'I have the book and it is fantastic. I have been following the flat tummy club now since the beginning of the year and it has transformed my tummy and other bits!! The book will stay by my side just to remind me what I have achieved and what I can achieve.'

'I love the book it was what my nutritionist advised me to do and now it is in print, Genius! I have had a wobble this lunch-time resorting to a sandwich for lunch totally unsatisfying and now reinforces that planning for wobbles and being fully supplied with good and loverly stuff even at work is the way forward. Going to put this lunchtime behind me and move on to some lovely miso salmon for dinner. Thanks for your sound and totally supportive book.'

"I'm now four weeks into the FTC and have lost 9lbs. I'm thrilled, and really motivated. I'm terrible at sticking to diets but here I am quite happily continuing. Best for me is that it seems to have stopped cravings and evened out my blood sugar levels. And going away or going out with friends for meals no longer spell diet disaster. I'll be 50 this year and at this rate I'm hoping to be in better shape at 50 than in my 40's. I've bought loads of diet books in my time but this is the only one I needed."

'Thank u sooo much Kate have bought your book and loving the read — got my big 50 bday approaching soon and this is definitely the way I want to spend the rest of my life.'

'I love simple food and enjoy what I eat so I am really excited about your book! Tonight we've had salmon teriyaki with green veg and rice. So yummy and so easy!'

'Got the book, how refreshingly different from other "diet" books! I am making small changes already and holidays are only 12 days away, hope I can continue (to a degree!) when I'm away. :-) Looking forward to my butternut squash soup for lunch and harissa chicken and cous cous for dinner!'

'I have fallen in love with the website and tips etc, even had poached egg on asparagus last night!'

'I brought your book yesterday and read up to week one and now off to Tesco to restock my cupboards!! I have even resisted a chocolate egg that my husband and sons were eating in front of me!! The best thing is I don't feel like I'm on a diet, I'm in control... Thanks for writing the book it's fabulous.'

'Got the book yesterday, read it avidly while travelling on the bus, started to plan where I need to make changes! Such a motivating, honest approach to a healthier lifestyle, not just losing weight. I am determined to get my body back!!'

'Here's to a new me! Already it makes so much sense.'

The Flat Tummy Club Diet

21 Days to a Flatter Tummy

Kate Adams

HODDER

First published in Great Britain in 2011 by Hodder & Stoughton
An Hachette UK company

This edition first published in 2012

1

A CIP catalogue record for this title is available from the British Library

ISBN 978 1 44470 851 6
Ebook ISBN 978 1 44470 852 3

Typeset in Plantin Light by Hewer Text UK Ltd, Edinburgh

Printed and bound by Clays Ltd, St Ives plc

Hodder & Stoughton policy is to use papers that are natural, renewable
and recyclable products and made from wood grown in sustainable forests.
The logging and manufacturing processes are expected to conform to
the environmental regulations of the country of origin.

Hodder & Stoughton Ltd
338 Euston Road
London NW1 3BH

www.hodder.co.uk

Although every effort has been made to ensure the contents of this book
are accurate, the information provided is not meant to take the place of
medical or nutrition advice from professionals. Please consult your physician
before starting a diet plan. The author cannot be held responsible for any
loss or claim arising out of the use or misuse of the suggestions made.

To the Adams Family

Contents

ACKNOWLEDGEMENTS

Thank you to my friends and family who supported me in my mad idea. Dawn and Hen have been my flat tummy partners in crime from day one, my sister Sam has been a real inspiration and my mum and dad ensure I always have something to write about, from Mum's walking journal to Dad's latest cooking adventure.

I owe great thanks to the entire team at Hodder, and in particular Nicky, Sarah, Emma and Kelly. You're a joy to work with. Thanks to Kay Halsey for very helpful and patient editing. And thank you to my agent Clare Hulton, who spotted my blog in the early days and 'just had a feeling'. Thanks to Anwen Hooson at Riot Communications for helping get us off the groud, and to Keith Wilson and Tom Gosling for my fabulous website.

Thank you to Elanor Wallis-Scott for the Flat Tummy Mummy exercises and for helping 'find my core'; you are a great teacher. And to Caroline, Camilla, Hugo, Rupert, Sara, Sam, Katy and Jacq for your recipe contributions. Thanks to Luzia for your lovely herb newsletters and teaching me why so much bread makes us bloated!

If you are an author I have worked with over the years and happen to be reading this book then thank you; my passion in life is to learn and so feel very lucky when I look back at the books I published and now to the books I help write.

My biggest thanks go to anyone who has ever stumbled upon the Flat Tummy Club and stuck around.

Every reasonable effort has been made to contact copyright holders, but if there are any errors or omissions, Hodder & Stoughton will be pleased to insert the appropriate acknowledgement in any subsequent printing of this publication.

Muriel Barbery, *The Elegance of the Hedgehog*; Gallic Books, 2008. Published originally under the title *L'Elegance du Herisson*, copyright © Editions GALLIMARD, Paris, 2006. Translation copyright © Europa Editions Inc. 2008.

James O. Prochaska, John C. Norcross, Carlo DiClemente, *Changing for Good*; Avon Books, 1998.

Alice Waters, *The Art of Simple Food*, Michael Joseph, 2008.

The National Weight Control Registry **www.nwcr.ws**

INTRODUCTION

*Eat the way you look at a beautiful picture or sing in a
beautiful choir.*

– Muriel Barbery, *The Elegance of the Hedgehog*

My Story

I used to publish diet books. Big, bestselling, blockbuster
diet books. And what happened? I put on over 2 stone and
developed a spare tyre around my middle . . . this is how I
lost it without losing my mind and how anyone can too,
living in the real world.

I had all the good intentions in the world and they were
always at their height on Sunday evenings. 'This week I'm
going on a health kick . . .' and then life just seemed to keep
getting in the way, usually by Tuesday. I had no excuses. I
was a health publisher, surrounded by the latest advice.
And yet, I was so wrapped up in deadlines and ambitions
that I forgot how much I love to feel energetic and full of
vitality. I fell into the trap of comforting stress with my
nemesis foods and alcohol. I picked from the buffet of diets

I had at my fingertips: low-carb worked for a while, until I could take life without bread no more, and I filled my cupboards with healthy foods that sat there staring at me.

I was frustrated that I could no longer fit into any of my clothes. My tummy had become a dreaded muffin top, which I guess is another sign that your jeans are the wrong size. I often felt bloated, sluggish and slow and remembered a few years before when I walked everywhere, was full of beans and felt great about myself and about life. When I tell friends now that I was more than 2 stone overweight, they often refuse to believe me.

'So where did you hide it?'

'Your scales must've been lying.'

'I just don't remember you putting on weight.'

Well, for me, the extra inches were pretty evenly distributed all over my body, from my thighs to my bum, my tummy and my arms. And I didn't gain weight quickly; over three years the pounds just crept on, very quietly and very gradually.

Many of us have a trigger when it comes to weight gain. It might be giving up smoking, never quite managing to shift the baby weight or letting stress get the better of us. For me the initial trigger was a fall down some stairs and a dislocated shoulder. Unfortunately I developed a frozen shoulder as a result and found it incredibly difficult to cook for a few months, plus I could only walk a little way before the deep ache in my shoulder set in. I had to resort to ready meals or picnic dinners and became quite sedentary (not to mention fed up).

My healthy habits slowly deserted me and even when my shoulder was back to normal, I didn't make an automatic return to lots of walking and healthy eating. I was in the cliché vicious circle as the lack of exercise and good food affected my energy and stress levels, both in the wrong direction, and the lack of energy meant I couldn't be bothered to go for my usual long walks at the weekend. I still indulged in edible treats; I just stopped burning them off.

Once you have got out of the habit of healthy living, it's no mean feat to start up again, especially for more than a couple of days. As my trousers started getting tighter and tighter and I went up a size, and then another, I would spend the weekends promising myself that this was the week I would change. But it just never got beyond the vague promises. I was continually disappointing myself and feeling like I had no willpower at all; I practically wrote myself off as just being weak.

So how *did* I make the change and see it through beyond the first few days, weeks and now years? Why did it work? What did I do? And why did I end up starting the Flat Tummy Club?

- I was honest with myself and with anyone who would listen
- I focused
- I made a plan
- I committed to the plan and found the time
- I used my brain and improved my knowledge
- I was optimistic and also realistic
- I dealt with my stress
- I ate delicious food
- I enjoyed myself
- I roped in a friend

All these steps just happen to be proven to help ensure successful weight loss that lasts. I pulled together all my favourite strands of knowledge from across my 10 years of health publishing and began to formulate a plan. I knew that buying a week's worth of healthy food and promising myself to exercise every day wasn't going to cut it, so I would have to do some preparation work first.

I started the first week with an exercise in honesty: keeping a full and complete food, drink and exercise diary the week before New Year. A friend joined me and in early January we went through our diaries, weighed ourselves and even took pictures. It was hilarious and a wake-up call – a good combination. It soon became clear what we each needed to do if we wanted to lose our tummies. I needed to replace the crisps, cheese and booze that had taken over my life and my friend needed to curb her comfort foods. We both needed to find the healthy foods we love and move a lot more.

I took up my own challenge and went for it. I planned that first week with military precision and when I did go out for meals, I scoured the menu for the healthiest options, often very pleasantly surprised as a result. I've still got my diary and I ate plenty of food, but it was all *real food*. I replaced sandwiches with soups, ate a lot of clementines and smoothies and I cooked easy, healthy dinners. I walked every day, whatever the weather. In a week I lost 7lbs of Christmas indulgence, which was just the motivation I needed to keep going, as well as finding it so much easier to get out of bed in the morning, feeling less stiff, far less bloated and about a million times better mid-afternoon.

Three months later, I had lost my initial 1½ stone target, another three months and another ½ stone. Over a year later and I am a walking cliché, but I feel so much better, more energized, more balanced. I'm back in my old jeans, 30 bags of sugar lighter and even feel good in a bikini!

First Days of the Flat Tummy Club

I started the Flat Tummy Club with my friend as a bit of a laugh, especially as everyone kept calling it the *Fat* Tummy Club by mistake. We had a founding membership of two, but as I told people what we were up to, friends started asking, 'Well, can I join?' We had created our very own mini 'slimming club' without having to go to the local community hall on a Monday evening.

I ventured into the world of Facebook and started emailing the Flat Tummy Club every week with a few tips, thoughts and recipes. One brave friend gave an anonymous review of having a colonic (see page 227), while another became my snack guru and 'Dawn's Banana Loaf' (see page 369) began its journey towards the cult status it enjoys today. A blog and website eventually followed, and now a book! The message from that first day, when my friend and I could hardly manage to take photos of each other for laughing, stays exactly the same . . .

Feel good, not guilty!

I'm one of those people who are pretty independent and happy in their own company, but there are times when a bit of friendly support is invaluable. I had felt bad about myself for years, but here I was, feeling great and having a laugh. Personally, I think it's incredibly easy to fall into putting on weight, but once you do so, it then gets wrapped up in all sorts of feelings of self-esteem, control and our sense of happiness. Everyone is different and we all have a compli-cated relationship both with food and with our health. I was out of balance and it's that sense of being level again that I cherish.

Going on a fad diet with weird rules could never have given me that balanced approach. I might've managed a couple of weeks and then what? Back to square one. I needed to embrace a healthier lifestyle full stop, one that two years later I'm still very happy to live.

Enough About Me, What About You?

The point of Flat Tummy Club is that it's about *you*. *The Flat Tummy Club Diet* helps you not only to get a flatter tummy, but stay at your happy, healthy weight – no counting calories or mung beans required (unless you like them).

There are some initial steps I take you through before you even change what's on your shopping list. We tackle the mind first, writing your own diary and using a simple questionnaire, so that you can recognize where your tummy came from and discover the impetus to stop vaguely promising yourself to eat less bread or go on a detox, and instead create a fully fledged plan.

We then create the practical plan, because all the research and my own experience show that preparation is the key to success. I am also here to help you stick to your plan and overcome the challenges: from getting home so late you just can't be bothered to cook to Monday mornings when you wonder if all this healthy living is really worth it. There are specific Flat Tummy tips, from Banish the Bloat (see page 129) to Flat Tummy teas, foods, Flat Tummy Workout exercises and restaurant know-how.

Thanks to everyone in the Flat Tummy Club, there are

anecdotes throughout that, if you are anything like me, you might just recognize, from sugar binges at the weekend to not knowing how to lose weight and cook for teenage children at the same time. And there's plenty of inspiration, from one woman who tried the Portuguese Chicken and Mint Soup (see page 278) and now makes it practically every week to another who simply started eating a healthy breakfast every day and hasn't looked back.

The beauty of *The Flat Tummy Club Diet* is that you get to make your own decisions and create your own simple plan, rather than try to follow a one-size-fits-all approach that however hard you try, you can't shoehorn into your daily life or that makes you feel you are on a depressing deprivation diet. With a few prompting questions, you will soon discover that *you know the answers* to how you can lose weight or stay slim because you know your body better than anyone else.

The key is to start with a positive and honest attitude. If you start to feel really good about yourself and put your health at the top of your agenda, then in turn the effect on those around you will be equally positive. I've also found that being positive about my health and fitness has had an amazing impact on my life in general – I'm more relaxed and optimistic, comfortable with myself and confident with others. That's why the Flat Tummy Club is a guilt-free zone, because if you lose weight from a negative starting point, it will never last.

I will help you put your plan into action, day by day for the first three weeks and with plenty of practical ideas and recipes for continuing for as long as you need to lose weight. My hope is that you will then discover changes that can last a lifetime, because they fit *your* life, rather than leaving you wondering what on earth to do once the sachets of 'diet soup' run out! It's all about being self-aware, maintaining a balance and continually firing up your passion for finding new foods, activities and healthy inspirations.

The Perfect Diet?

Every diet book you pick up will claim to have something that is missing from all the other diet books before, and I can vouch for the fact that there have been many, many before. Why is it that we are so obsessed with finding the perfect diet and yet as a nation seem to find it incredibly hard to lose weight, and especially to keep the weight off once we've lost it? Why did my friend, who is the healthiest eater I know, order a raw food diet book to lose her post-baby tummy when she already knew exactly what to do? How did I manage to put on a couple of extra stone when I was surrounded by diet advice?

Has 'Nutrition' Gone Mad?

A casual look through my 'diet and nutrition' bookshelf, which exists purely for professional purposes of course, reveals that the search for the perfect diet has taken many turns over the years, decades and even centuries.

There are a couple of books telling me to eat mainly protein and I'll lose weight quickly and healthily, while books based on research of the healthiest societies in the world urge me to eat less meat and more vegetables. One book champions raw food, while another tells me raw food is harder to digest. Fat is evil, oh hang on, fat is essential. Fasting is my saviour, no, wait, eating little and often is the answer to all my weight loss prayers.

And so it goes on. Even my friends, on discovering that Flat Tummy Club was being turned into a book, all urged me to 'tell them what to do'. But what exactly is the right thing to do? I started to panic that my own weight loss wasn't scientifically proven. I didn't know if a carrot contained more nutrients than a squash per gram and hadn't I read somewhere about a diet that banned all orange foods anyway? It was the same when it came to exercise. During the same weekend, I read one article in the paper about exercise having no effect on weight loss and another saying that exercise was an essential part of successful weight loss!

If you have formed the habit of checking on every new diet that comes along, you will find that, mercifully, they all blur together, leaving you with only one definite piece of information: French-fried potatoes are out.

– Jean Kerr

Why Is Losing Weight So Hard Anyway?

In theory losing weight and staying slim should be the easiest thing in the world – eat a healthy diet and exercise, right? But if it were that easy, there'd be no such phrase as 'yo-yo' dieting and the government wouldn't spend millions of pounds and thousands of thinking hours trying to make the nation healthier. There are other factors at play and it's worth exploring a bit of the background to understand why diet has become such a weighty issue.

The challenges of the modern diet

Food is intrinsically something we have a natural relationship with, but in the past 150 years or so it has become highly industrialized and commoditized, in many cases almost beyond recognition. It's not just that grains are so much easier to grow than vegetables, but when you process them you can turn them into such an array of profitable 'foods' that can be marketed into our consciousness; it's no wonder that the green leafies start to lose their appeal.

In nature, foods give us signals that they are ready to eat and at their most nutritious through our sense of smell, sight, touch and taste. Just think of the sweet smell and slight give of a ripe melon, or that wonderful aroma of vine tomatoes that are deep red, firm to the touch and sweet on the tongue.

But now we are surrounded by artificial flavours and artificial foods that confuse the natural relationship. We are born with a tendency to like sweet foods, but that is so we eat fruit and vegetables when they are ready and good for us and avoid the berries that are poisonous. When faced with the array of *unnaturally* sweet foods on the supermarket shelves, our inner sweet detector can't tell the difference. And of course, these are the foods we see most often promoted and on offer. We notice fruit and vegetables in big end-of-aisle promotions during January, but the rest of the year it's 48 packets of crisps, kids' cereals coated in sugar and giant bottles of fizzy drinks.

Whole foods have become increasingly refined. White flour lasts so much longer on the shelf that it has made white bread a staple available to all, no matter that the goodness found in the germ of the wheat has been removed to make this possible. Sugar is refined so much to make it white that it is literally a shock to our system. And healthy complex carbohydrates have been turned into simple carbohydrates, which release energy so quickly that our body just stores the overflow as fat.

Nature and nurture

It's a relief to me to realize that, like just about everything in life, weight gain is something that is born of both nature and nurture. Some people really do have a tendency to put on weight *in certain circumstances*. And that's where our culture plays such an important role, both in terms of the wider society, but also our own individual or family culture, which we do have some control over.

You can see this being played out right now in the shopping malls of Portugal. The more traditional cultural diet of Portugal is very simple – fish or meat with vegetables, marinades, spices, and fish and rice stews. It's delicious and while Portuguese people might not all be skinny, they look pretty good to me. But literally in the last few years as shopping malls have sprung up along the Algarve, the favoured restaurant of increasing numbers of young Portuguese is the burger bar, completely alien to the traditional culture, but shiny and new and a statement of youth. The 'nurture' part of the equation is changing and upsetting the balance; obesity is on the rise.

From the car to the office

In America, it's often impossible to just step out of the door and go for a walk. I lived in Kansas for a year of university with a couple of English friends and I'll never forget the evening we tried to walk to the furniture rental store. Halfway there the pavement literally ran out and we had no choice but to inch our way along a highway; there wasn't even a verge we could walk along. The people in their cars looked at us with expressions either asking if we were OK or were we mad. Even here in the UK it's easy to go for days at a time driving to work and back with the quickest of walks at lunchtime to find a sandwich. And walking takes time we think we don't have; life is a rush.

Because of this industrialization of food, combined with our workplace culture becoming more sedentary for such a large majority of us, it's easy to get out of balance with nature when it comes to food, eating and health. We are a consumer society now and the vast majority of foods you see advertised on the television are processed and bear little resemblance to anything found down on the farm. It's very easy to sit in an office all day, chat over a cup of tea and a few biscuits and drive or catch the bus home. Feeling mentally shattered, we then lack the willpower to exercise or cook from scratch, but instead reach for the wine and something convenient, often processed. Things are not set up well right now for us to find it easy to enjoy a healthy lifestyle or, if we need to, lose weight. It takes a concerted effort, but once you make the initial push, I've found it to be liberating, which is why I'm so thrilled you have even picked up this book. Self-awareness and a *desire to be healthy* are the first and ever so crucial steps.

How Is Flat Tummy Club Different?

As I explored my shelf of diets, there was something I kept coming back to, and it had nothing to do with scientific studies or following some kind of regime for the rest of my life. It was that the Flat Tummy Club had allowed me to break free of my bad habits and embrace healthy eating and healthy living for what it was – feeling good. I hadn't become a food saint, but I was back in balance with what's right for my body and my wellbeing. And I'd made a conscious decision to do that rather than following some directions on the packet. I'd put all the pieces of the weight loss puzzle together rather than picking from one or another as I'd tried to do over the years.

For me this is the key difference with Flat Tummy Club – it's a slightly old-fashioned word, but it's a holistic approach that first gets your brain and self-awareness in gear, empowers you with knowledge about food and healthy living, prepares you for change, jump starts your plan and finally enthuses you to keep going! Because once you are self-aware, you can recognize when you go off track and tweak your lifestyle accordingly, rather than play a game of snakes and ladders.

This book is all about creating a practical plan to follow, and follow to the letter for a good while until your bad habits begin to loosen their grip on your willpower. But this time *you* are going to be the person who determines the plan. You're the one who is going to use all the in-depth knowledge you already have about yourself to eat vegetables you like, rather than because they are on a list of 'all-you-can-eat' foods. If you work in an office, I'm not going to saddle you with trying to work out how to make a smoothie for your mid-morning snack when you know you can eat a pot of yoghurt, drink a cup of miso soup or just go ahead and have a banana instead.

For me, being active goes hand in hand with eating more healthily too, and whatever the latest study says, you can be sure another one will pop up saying the opposite. What does your common sense tell you? What does your own experience tell you? When I'm exercising regularly, I don't seem to need to worry too much about what I eat and I tend to have extra energy to cook from scratch more often, I generally have less guilt about what I'm eating. It's a win-win situation.

Many diets either want you to think yourself slim and forget about what you eat or give you a scientifically proven diet regime to follow religiously, but not really consider why you are doing it in the first place. Within the food-based diets, there always has to be a gimmick, from cayenne pepper to lemon juice, raw food to macrobiotic. Within the 'thinking' diets, it's no surprise that the most popular are those that promise to do it for you at the flick of a switch. I realized when I decided to make my own plan that I needed to cater to both my mind, which had become rather lazy and seemed to constantly be making bad food choices, and my taste buds, which needed firing up. And what was the point in eating well while being a couch potato? Surely being healthy meant connecting up all the dots. I could use my brain to convince myself to eat porridge in the morning, which in turn inspired me to make my own compote. After a delicious breakfast, I then had the energy to walk an hour to work, which meant I arrived refreshed and ready for the day.

The Flat Tummy Club Challenge

I am not a nutritionist. I am not a personal trainer or a scientist. I am a normal person who will eat the local doughnuts dipped in hot chocolate sauce while on holiday in Spain because hours later, I'll be choosing the freshest fruit, vegetables and just-caught fish from the market to enjoy for dinner. I do have this 'thing' about real food and I don't understand why it's not the trendiest way to lose inches and stay at a happy weight. I think it's because, understandably, we want losing weight to be as easy as possible and we've all grown up with a food industry that tells us the easiest and most convenient foods are the ones that are processed – that are made for us. These foods have even taken over the meaning of the words 'fast' and 'convenience'. What's faster than slicing open an avocado and eating it? What's more convenient than a banana?

It's always been a bit of a mission of mine to get the word out that healthy eating isn't boring. Somehow the lines have been drawn between 'real' food and 'diet' food and it has left a huge legacy of confusion and disempowerment over our health. We lose the weight and then don't know how on earth to return to a happy, balanced, enjoyable way of eating. We worry that a slice of bread will signal our immediate downfall; we scrutinize menus trying to count up the calories or carbs, rather than looking for the freshest, most delicious dishes. In the Flat Tummy Club, we look for those freshest, most delicious dishes and I know it sounds on the dangerous verge of smug, but I'd even venture to say that losing weight can be enjoyable and inspire you to discover new foods and try new things. It doesn't have to be antisocial, depressing or boring.

FLAT TUMMY CLUB MEMBERSHIP BENEFITS

More energy
Less bloating
Fewer hangovers
Better sleep
Feeling positive
Less stiffness
No afternoon slumps
Less stress
Less anxiety

2

GET READY...

How to Change
We know it's good, but that doesn't mean we like it

I think that successful change can be encouraged by external forces, for example whether I inspire you enough to write your food diary (coming up on page 26), create your plan and go for it. But for there to be lasting change, it has to come from within.

I really like the Stages of Change Model, originally developed in the late 1970s by James Prochaska and Carlo DiClemente at the University of Rhode Island. They were studying how some people were able to give up smoking, but the model also applies to all sorts of behaviour involving personal change, including weight loss. I think it helps to explain why there is no one magic diet to end all diets.

The theory is that we don't change instantly, but we progress through a series of six steps. And the cliché is true that other people can't force you to change, you can only move through the steps at your own pace through inner control.

The Stages of Change Model

1. Pre-contemplation (you don't yet know or acknowledge there is anything to change)
2. Contemplation (you acknowledge there is a problem, but you're not sure you want to change or you don't feel ready)
3. Preparation (you set your intention and work out how you're going to change)
4. Action (actual change)
5. Maintenance
6. Relapse

Pre-Contemplation

As G.K. Chesterton wrote, 'It isn't that they can't see the solution. It is that they can't see the problem.' Pre-contemplation is really another term for denial. We're just not aware of there being anything we need or want to change – quite frankly, we're just not that interested! If you bought this book yourself, then you've moved beyond the pre-contemplation stage by that very act of awareness and a willingness to make a change. But perhaps a friend or loved one recommended the book and you're not really sure why you're even reading it? Or you bought the book ages ago in a random moment of action, but then it sat on the shelf gathering dust. The holiday you wanted to get in shape for has long been and gone, but you've now decided to take a look and see what this Flat Tummy Club is all about. Well, get ready for some contemplation . . .

Contemplation

Things are still not 100 per cent hunky-dory in the contemplation stage when it comes to making a lifestyle change.

This is where we ruminate about whether we can really be bothered to put the effort in? Ask ourselves if giving up crisps or wine is worth it? Does it actually matter if we lose weight or not in the grand scheme of things? Before you think I've gone mad, I'm not trying to put you off, but I'm just being completely honest – after all I had all these thoughts myself. What I do hope is that I can inspire and encourage you to move along to the next stage a bit quicker than I managed. I contemplated losing weight and getting healthy for a good couple of years. At least I had moved on from being in oblivious pre-contemplation, but the problem was that I became stuck in contemplation, and every time I asked myself on a Sunday evening to get ready for a health kick, it turned out I couldn't be bothered. I was engaging in wishful thinking, a classic obstacle to action.

There are certain things that help to tip the balance in favour of making a definite decision to change, and without even realizing it, I used these tools to initiate my own change with great success.

Consciousness-raising

The best way to create a strong foundation for change is to raise your self-awareness and also arm yourself with plenty of knowledge, both about yourself and about healthy living.

I've read lots of diets that say 'throw away the scales' as they quite rightly don't want us to become unhealthily obsessed with our weight. Before I embarked on my own weight loss plan, I hadn't stepped on the scales in about five years. Of course I knew I'd put on weight because none of my trousers fitted, but stepping onto my friend's scales meant that, for once and for all, I couldn't deny the facts any longer. And it might not be a 100 per cent foolproof method for finding out if you are overweight, but there was no denying my BMI (see page 82) was on the wrong end of the scale – it was unhealthy. Writing a food and exercise diary was also an important consciousness-raising step. I had to make a concerted effort to be 100 per cent honest with myself and include everything that passed my lips so that I could take a good look at my lifestyle. After all, what was the point in continuing to con myself – I'd never lose weight that way!

In addition to the indisputable facts, I also spent time consciousness-raising in a way that properly engaged how I felt. My body confidence was at an all time low, and I'm not talking about an 'I'm so wonderful, my body is amazing' type of body confidence, but the one that simply makes you feel comfortable in your own skin. As the mighty Gok would say, you certainly don't have to be slim to have body confidence, but for me it was a question of health. I didn't like that I was eating rubbish and feeling stressed and bloated. I wanted to regain my sense of vitality – the inner healthy me.

In Food Facts (see page 41) I will arm you with healthy eating knowledge so that you can see clearly what a balanced diet really looks like, both if you need to lose weight and when you want to stay slim for the everyday longer term. I've also included tips on exercise (see page 99) and if, like me, you're not the most confident of cooks, there's plenty of healthy cooking inspiration and lots of easy recipes (see page 259).

Preparation

Preparation is our best friend when it comes to making a successful change. As a part of this stage it's vital to address any potential obstacles. We have to be honest with ourselves about what we're giving up and feel confident that the benefits outweigh the effort that will be required. We also have to be careful we don't build a shaky case for change that can be blown over like a house of cards. We have to commit, prioritize our decision and the efforts we'll be putting into it, take it step by step, announce our commitment to the world (or at least to our friends and family) and put together a plan, from writing out our shopping list to putting exercise in our diary to looking ahead at the week's various challenges and thinking through how we're going to tackle them successfully.

Action

The part you've been waiting for, the action stage, is where you 'simply' replace your previous behaviour with healthier alternatives. This is the part that often lasts about three days before you lapse (see below). But if you've built a strong enough case for change in your mind and prepared on a practical level, then you stand a much greater chance of seeing it through. I think this explains why women who are getting married are often so self-disciplined when it comes to fitting into their wedding dress. It's a once-in-a-lifetime day and so the motivation and commitment are plentiful, plus they are in full planning mode anyway. It also explains why so many New Year resolutions fall by the wayside within a few days or weeks. Often we'll start a health kick on 1 January, but we've done no thinking time or preparation in the run up – we've been too busy eating and drinking and being merry. It's fine if we were slim before Christmas and just need to lose those couple of extra pounds, but if we want to lose more than our Christmas pudding weight, then launching straight into a detox once the celebrations are over won't be all that likely to last us through to the summer.

I did start my road to a Flat Tummy in January, but I also spent Christmas gearing up for the change I was going to be making. My food diary was embarrassing: every chocolate and every nut was noted down. But I didn't feel bad because I was starting to feel really confident that I would follow through with my healthy plans. And as ever with these things, just the act of writing a food diary did help me reach for fewer chocolates and try and stick to very small pieces of cake!

Maintenance

Maintenance is a word that anyone who has been on any kind of diet will be extremely familiar with. It's the Holy Grail of dieting, how to keep it going for life. If we make lifestyle changes that feel good and that we start to really enjoy, then we are much more likely to maintain them. It's also important to be realistic in our goals and not expect ourselves to never let a cake pass our lips again. What we can do is to create a healthy balance. We can tip the odds in our favour and make enough good choices and develop enough healthy habits that mean we don't yo-yo. The key is to develop an easy and natural relationship with food and keep our self-awareness strong.

Relapse

It's human to lapse. We're faced with challenges and choices every day and we won't make the right decisions 100 per cent of the time – life would be boring if we did – so don't set that goal because you're just not being fair on yourself.

I think when it comes to food, it's a question of how you define a mini or full relapse. For example, I don't eat now how I ate in the first few weeks when I began to lose the weight. I could feel like a failure every time I have a croissant, but because I walk so much during the week and eat healthy food 90 per cent of the time, I thoroughly enjoy the odd croissant.

For me, I feel like I've relapsed when I haven't made any conscious decision about what I'm about to eat, but just mindlessly choose something unhealthy that I don't even really want. The trick with these relapses is to not let it lead to more, but rather to go straight back to contemplation, pass quickly through preparation, action and back into maintenance, or 'happy balance' mode.

I like the Stages of Change Model because it explains why we often feel such failures when we give up on a diet or exercise regime quickly, whereas it's really because we never thought it through properly. If we try and force change when we've just started contemplating and we're not all that convinced the benefits are worth the effort, it is no wonder we have so many aborted attempts. Perhaps I didn't need to spend two years in contemplation, but once I got to stage three, my determination was very strong.

As you read through the book, you should naturally move through the Stages of Change. Do come back to this chapter for extra oomph if you hit a wobble patch. You may need to remind yourself why being healthy and slim is worth making a change for, whether big or small, to see yourself full of energy. You may have tried to dive straight in without planning and struggled at the first challenge, say, an invitation to the pub or a big piece of a colleague's birthday cake. Don't berate yourself and give up for good, tomorrow is a new healthy day.

Start Today

Rather than make you read through half a book of background information that I hope will persuade you to my way of thinking, I'm going to ask you to get stuck in right now. There are two things I want you to do:

1. Start writing your own food and exercise diary.
2. Get to the heart of why you put the weight on.

Through being completely honest with yourself, you raise your self-awareness and begin to strengthen your resolve. Even if you are slim and just picked up this book to tone up in time for a holiday or to lose your pot belly and simply want me to tell you what to eat and how many crunches to do, this exercise will help you notice the little changes you can implement to make a real difference that lasts beyond your holiday.

The key is to be 100 per cent honest, so carry a little notebook around or use your diary as it's much harder to remember everything at the end of the day. You will start to notice things pretty quickly: habits, mindless eating or a tendency to have second portions. Add as much detail as you can:

- Whether you only feel human after your first cup of coffee
- Where you get lunch
- Which meals are cooked from scratch
- Anything you grab on the run during the day
- Do you eat at your desk?
- Are you a constant snacker or do you save yourself for big dinners that leave you feeling a bit stuffed?
- What is your 'nemesis' – the food, or foods, that you just can't seem to eat in moderation?
- What are your triggers for eating foods you know are unhealthy?
- How much time in the day do you spend sitting versus walking?

KATE'S FAT TUMMY DIARY

On rising: Cup of tea

Breakfast: Raisin toast with banana

Mid-morning: 2 cups of coffee (white Americano)

Lunch: Chicken salad sandwich and crisps (637 calories for a lunch that made me suffer the dreaded afternoon slump)

Mid-afternoon: Cup of tea and a couple of choc biscuits (to counter that afternoon slump)

Dinner: Leek and St Agur risotto (not incredibly unhealthy, but portion control non-existent) and cheese and biscuits

Drinks: Glass of water, 2 big glasses of wine, herbal tea

Exercise: ½ hour walking on the way home: packet of crisps (a habit I got into)

How do I feel? Shattered

My typical day was a bit of a rollercoaster with two coffees in quick succession, up then down; a very uninspiring lunch; hardly any water/herbal tea and that dreadful feeling in the afternoon when you can hardly keep your eyes open. I also got into the habit of pouring a glass of wine every evening. It became a symbolic end to the day at work, but depleted my energy even more, meaning my evenings were usually spent as a couch potato. With just half an hour of walking during the whole day, I felt sluggish and lazy. All a bit stodgy really.

For some people, being honest about the exact number of biscuits eaten in a day is a tough challenge. For others, like me, it's being straight up about exactly how much alcohol we consume in a day and, even more revealing, in a week. The number of units recommended as being healthy for the average woman to consume in a week is 14, and no more than 3 in a day. For men, it is 21 in a week, and no more than 4 in a day. Put in real terms, sharing a bottle of wine between two is the equivalent of each person drinking just under 5 units each, more than the recommended daily amount for both men and women. A pint of 5% lager is 2.84 units and there are 1.4 units in an average pub measure (35ml) of spirits. You can see how easily it adds up. A healthy consumption would look like a small glass of red with supper each night or a couple of small glasses three nights a week.

Writing a food, drink and exercise diary is so helpful because it tests your honesty and engages your brain. It's fascinating to me how hard it is to write down every single thing you eat and drink in the day, but I think once I did it, I almost felt relieved because it became so obvious what I needed to do to make a difference. I also stopped mindlessly eating so much because I had to remember everything I was eating – I had to start paying attention.

This is how the Flat Tummy Club Diet diary tends to look in contrast.

KATE'S FLAT TUMMY DIARY

On rising: Herbal tea or lemon juice and hot water

Breakfast: Porridge with a little honey/compote or natural yoghurt and berries with a sprinkle of granola

Snack: An Innocent smoothie, a cup of miso soup or a clementine

Lunch: A BIG soup with flatbread

Snack: A strip of dark chocolate or a couple of fruity or seeded oatcakes

Dinner: Lemon and Ginger Salmon (see page 313) with stir-fried pak choy and spring onions

Drinks: Green tea, peppermint tea, nettle tea, water with a squeeze of lime

Exercise: A walk before work and at lunch time, 10 minutes of Flat Tummy Workout.

How do I feel? Healthy, more energetic and focused, paying more attention to what I'm eating and as a result enjoying food more

Notice how you feel when you are eating. When do you feel really great and when do pangs of guilt rise up? Do you savour your food or hoover it up while watching television?

It's a good idea to get to the bottom of why you put the weight on in the first place. My mum just assumed she was getting older and a bit fatter, but when she started to think about it honestly, she realized that she had been walking less and less over time, initially because of a toe problem, but had then found it harder to walk because she had less puff as she had put on weight. Mum could easily have just thrown up her hands and declared her weight gain was therefore none of her fault, but the thing is, it's not about finding fault or blame. It's about realizing that you can often stop these negative cycles and turn them around. For my mum, the combination of realizing where a lot of her weight gain originated and also taking a look at what she was eating, meant she recognized what she could do to start making a difference. After all, she could walk 'a bit' and could therefore build up gradually over time. And that was the first step that triggered a domino effect. By walking more, she felt better about herself and found her need for comforting cakes also began to diminish. She didn't set ridiculous goals to be the same size as when she was 20 (more on that later) but is, quite frankly, a new woman. On a holiday to Italy with my dad, they rang me on my birthday. 'Kate, Kate, we're having a fabulous time. We're walking before breakfast, picking figs and being really good, apart from the Prosecco!'

You Are What You Think

The belly is the giver of genius.
– Persius (Roman satirical poet)

It's interesting that we have so many phrases that show the connection between our minds and our digestion.

- Food for thought
- I'll digest that
- Something to chew on
- Gut instinct

And now science is backing up this link, which somehow we've always known, with hard evidence. The connection goes both ways. Our emotions affect our digestion, especially anger, anxiety and upset. Our brain sends direct messages to the stomach when we are hungry, triggering stomach juices in preparation for digesting what we're about to eat. And the health of our digestion also has an impact on how we are feeling. People with very sensitive tummies or with irritable bowel syndrome (IBS) are often very sensitive in general.

I have never had terrible digestion, but I definitely feel the difference when it is a bit sluggish or sensitive versus when it's strong. It doesn't seem fair because this tummy–brain connection can easily send you into a bit of a negative cycle: you feel tense or stressed, which makes your digestion struggle to function really well, and in turn you don't get so much nutrition or energy from food and consequently start to feel a bit lethargic or tired. This makes the stress worse, you then crave sugary fixes that put strain on your digestion, and so on.

The good news is that you can equally create a positive cycle. I ate fantastically healthy food when I initially lost weight that clearly helped with my digestion. My energy levels picked up as a result and I started to feel more confident and relaxed, which in turn kept my tummy happy. Because I was feeling more balanced in more ways than one, I truly discovered that my cravings for sugar, salt and alcohol began to fade. Now when I detect the early signs of stress, I reach for foods that are easy on my digestion, like porridge, soup and the miracle that is Congee (see page 233).

As one Flat Tummy Club member said, you have to be 'in the mood' to be healthy and take a very conscious decision to make room in your life for it. Think of all the extremely good reasons for taking care of your body and your mind, both for you and also those close to you. I can vouch that living more healthily literally changes your life for the better, which I realize makes me sound evangelical, but when I compare how I feel now to when I was unnecessarily stressed, tired all the time and lacking in confidence, I can see it was worth making the change.

Paying Attention

When you are in the process of breaking bad habits and creating new ones, or training your willpower (see page 36), you do need to focus on the job in hand and use your mind as a tool. I like to think of this as mindfulness about what we choose to eat and then our actual experience of eating – as we think about the flavours, how the dish was created and how much we like it.

There was a brilliant experiment conducted by Brian Wansink where he revealed just how mindless we can be when it comes to eating. He had two groups: one was given a bowl of soup in a normal bowl, the other group was given a bowl of soup, but without them knowing the bowls could be continually refilled from the bottom. The second group ate a whopping 75 per cent more soup than the control group, without even realizing.

It was Professor Tanya Byron, the lovely and brilliant psychologist, who gave me some fantastic advice once: that it's not just 'you are what you eat', but 'you are what you *think*'. It's invaluable to remember that losing weight, and indeed getting a Flat Tummy, isn't just about doing five different types of crunches or eating three amazing fat-burning foods or hypnotizing yourself – it's putting together what we eat, do, think and feel and realizing that they all interlink and benefit each other.

Top tips

- Your tummy sends messages to your brain to signal that you are full, but unfortunately there is a bit of a time delay thanks to your digestion. If you stop eating when you are two-thirds full, then in a few minutes you will realize that you've actually had enough.

- Don't go shopping when you are hungry as the tummy–brain connection means you end up buying far more, and less healthy, food than you need.
- Along the same theme, don't turn up to a restaurant starving hungry as you will struggle to make good choices from the menu and will eat all the bread.
- Don't eat and work at the same time as using your brain will use up energy needed for efficient digestion. You won't absorb all the nutrition from your food and you may well feel tired later and in need of a pick-me-up.

Clearing Out Your Mental Clutter

We'll be having a kitchen detox later (see page 111), but it's also incredibly helpful if we can clear out our mental clutter every now and again too. If we can embrace a healthy change for both body and mind, then we're all the stronger for it. Make a fresh start with your relationship with food, but rather than ignore your niggles and issues, bring them out and think them, even talk them, through. Write your feelings down on paper. Be clear as crystal on why you want to be healthy and slim!

Feeling Good, Not Guilty

This is about as close as I come to making promises with the Flat Tummy Club, because I know that false promises are worse than no promises at all. But one thing that Flat Tummy Club definitely is, is optimistic. Because I'm a Virgo, and because unchecked optimism has been proven to be rather unhelpful in the successful achievement of goals, I also add a dash of realism to the optimism. There's no point seeing yourself as Angelina or Brad if you have no idea how to get started or how to tackle all the challenges that come your way as a part of daily life. But optimism and positive thoughts definitely have their benefits when combined with a step-by-step plan. I remember the stop-smoking guru extraordinaire Allen Carr saying that stopping smoking isn't about 'giving up', it's about the freedom to be a non-smoker. I used this tip when I first started to lose my excess pounds, focusing on all the healthy foods and herbal teas that I knew I liked or wanted to try, rather than mourning the loss of pain au chocolat. This has helped hugely in maintaining my weight loss. I don't have to go for the rest of my life feeling horrible pangs of guilt every time I do now look at a pain au chocolat. And I quite happily eat them every now and then because I'm back in control of my diet and my lifestyle.

In many cultures, the enjoyment of food is intrinsic to healthy eating. Just think of the Italians or the Greeks. In China there isn't even really a word for calories, and in Chinese medicine nutrition, it is said that enjoying the food we eat even makes it more nutritious, as we fire up our stomach juices with anticipation and relish.

A smiling face is half the meal.
Latvian proverb

Willpower – What Is It and Can I Get More of It?

You will, you will, you will . . .

From a personal point of view, I know that willpower is a fickle thing. One day, it's a trusty companion by your side as you choose soup and a salad for lunch and go home to make a lovely supper of baked salmon and steamed veggies. The next day, it's nowhere to be seen as you declare 'sod it' when the chocolate biscuits get offered round with afternoon tea and pour yourself a big glass of wine as soon as you set foot in the kitchen when you get home.

What exactly happens between the steamed veggies and the best part of a bottle of wine or packet of digestives? Why does our willpower to be healthy seem to come and go so easily and why is it that we find comfort in the very things that are bad for us? Are there ways that we can strengthen our willpower, or at least be prepared for the inevitable lapses?

The area of our brain responsible for willpower has many other things to take care of, including keeping us focused, solving certain problems and looking after short-term memory. If we ask it to do too much, then willpower just throws up its hands and gives up. If you've spent a long day at work solving problems, exercising your willpower to keep your cool in a meeting and generally using your brain a lot, then you literally run out of self-control by the time you get home and reach for whatever comforting food or drink you can lay your hands on.

It's therefore important while you are losing weight or developing healthy habits that you don't tempt fate and make it easy to give in to the cravings that will hit you when you're tired and stressed from a long day. Prepare lots of healthy and comforting food at the weekend, like big hearty soups and stews that you can reheat in minutes. For me, if there was a big packet of crisps in my cupboard I would eat it at the first opportunity, usually with a sandwich, and that would be dinner. So I did a big spring clean of my fridge and cupboards and filled them with good foods that I could either prepare lovingly or very quickly at the end of a hard day. I would also take time to relax on my commute home rather than continue working on the train and so further deplete the willpower reserves. And I started walking to and from the train station, about 45 minutes each way, morning and evening. Initially, of course, I did this for the exercise, but the added benefit was that I'd actually find the walk refreshing in a gentle, relaxing way at the end of the day. It was almost like a meditation as I'd breathe deeply and let the stresses and strains of the day fade away. By the time I'd get home, the urge to eat crisps and drink wine had faded too.

In other studies, blood sugar levels have also been shown to affect willpower, i.e. willpower requires energy. If you try and lose weight by missing meals, or you forget to eat because you're so busy, then your degree of self-control starts to diminish. If you're anything like me, then you turn into a bit of a crazed monster when your blood sugar drops too low and either start demanding food immediately from anyone in your vicinity or you just start snapping people's heads off for no good reason. When you've reached this point you know your willpower is no match for the monster and you grab the sweetest fix you can find. This is another reason it's so good to always keep your healthy snacks close at hand. My mantra is that a healthy balance in all aspects of our lifestyle is the goal, so it makes sense that keeping blood sugar levels on an even keel is so important when it comes to weight loss, particularly weight loss around the tummy.

Likewise, getting a good night's sleep powers up your willpower and studies have also shown that compromised sleep hinders fat loss in people trying to lose weight, plus less sleep makes us more hungry. Another interesting find has been in studying children who are able to resist one marshmallow for long enough to get a second. Hands up if that would include you? Then you have a head start when it comes to willpower. The trick is in distracting the mind, so rather than fixate on the marshmallow, the children sing songs or look at other things to take their mind off the temptation. This explains why I think of boredom as sugar's best friend and why I had so many baths in the first few weeks of losing the weight.

Surround yourself with people and things that make you feel good to boost your willpower. I have a friend who introduced me to a kickboxing workout class. It might not be the first thing she wants to do every Monday evening, but she's gone through the habit barrier and now just goes as a matter of course. If I had tried to start going to a new workout class purely under my own steam, to be honest I'd have given up, probably before I'd even started.

What's Your Motivation?

Overcoming an apparent lack of willpower can be done with the right motivation. Often it's just a case of needing enough oomph to get over the hump and then things get back on track. Exercise is the prime example of this. I don't know many people who run out of the door joyous at the sheer thought of going for a jog. Yes, they do exist, but they are few and far between. For most of us mortals, we have to use all the motivation tricks in the book to get ourselves started, but once we have, we feel great and can't think what all the fuss was about.

Motivation that works tends to be both manageable and meaningful. That's why we keep things incredibly simple at the Flat Tummy Club. It's important to spend time focusing on why you want to make a change. I realized after losing weight and keeping it off that my inner resolve was pretty strong because I'd taken a good look in the mirror and declared enough was truly enough. By combining that resolve with a carefully constructed plan of action, which I knew would fit simply into my life and wasn't unrealistic, I made it that much easier to get through the times when my willpower deserted me. I literally took it one day at a time, but also planned ahead and focused on the long-term benefits I'd enjoy. It's a powerful combination.

The great news is that when we do manage to use our willpower to overcome a challenge, like a craving for a comforting piece of chocolate cake, the benefits act like a ripple effect into all sorts of different areas. For example, people who create a healthy habit like going to an exercise class once a week will often become tidier, cook more, watch the television a bit less and do the washing up more! I can personally testify to the washing up part of that last sentence. And you can practise building up your willpower with anything you like, it doesn't have to just be about diet or exercise, but as your willpower improves, so will your consumption of vegetables.

Food Facts

I am not a dietician or nutritionist, so I'm just as curious as the next person about whether it's true that eating grapefruit shrinks your stomach or why on earth a mixture of maple syrup and cayenne pepper might promote weight loss. We are bombarded with weird and wonderful nutritional information every day and it can get confusing.

Did You Know?

1. You are at a higher risk of type 2 diabetes if your waist is 31.5 inches or over for Asian women, 33 inches for white and black women, 35 inches or over for Asian men and 37 inches or over for white and black men.
2. Being overweight or obese is likely to increase your risk of heart disease, whether you're an apple or a pear.
3. Green tea raises your metabolism but, before you get too excited, only by the equivalent of about 70 calories a day if you drink 5 cups.
4. Some carbohydrates are positively good for you.
5. Some fats are *essential*.
6. Lean protein keeps you fuller for longer per calorie than carbohydrates.

7. Soup also keeps your tummy satisfied for longer than if you were to eat the solid ingredients separately.
8. There appears to be no evidence that grapefruit shrinks your stomach or burns fat. It's still very good for you, it just doesn't have magic powers.
9. Technically, bananas are a herb.
10. The origins of the cabbage soup diet are unknown and no one claims responsibility.

This is how the average UK daily diet is broken down:

UK food consumption data

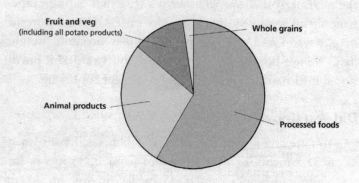

Using data from the 'National Diet Nutrition Survey Year 1 Report 2008/2009', Food Standards Agency.

When you see this, it doesn't take a PhD to work out why we are struggling to stay slim as a nation.

Calories

Yawn. Well, I might want to fight it with every big bone in my body, but it is worth keeping a gentle eye out for calories because if we consume too many that contain too little nutrition, then we put on weight. Personally, I think a life spent calculating calories or counting points would be miserable in the long term – where's the passion for food in that? What you can do is develop a general awareness of which foods contain very little nutrition for their calorie value and implement that knowledge in your cooking, shopping and restaurant ordering.

Here are a few tips worth remembering

- Fresh vegetables are low in calories and high in nutrition, so pack them into your daily diet. The leafy kinds are top of the tree.
- Eat two or three portions of any fresh fruit a day and you needn't worry about the calories.
- Dried fruit contains far more calories per gram than fresh fruit. It's a great snack, but this info is handy to be aware of.
- Refined sugary or starchy foods are often high in calories and aren't that satisfying per calorie, a bit of a no-win situation.
- Even essential fats (see page 50) are high in calories, so remember these are rich foods that are best in moderation.
- Get the most out of your calories. Eating 1500 calories worth of chocolate biscuits just isn't the same as 1500 calories worth of natural foods.
- The figure to look out for on food labels is 'kcal' and not 'kJ'. KJs are a smaller unit of energy than kcal (1kcal = 4.184kJ). When recommended calorie intakes are quoted, these are usually done so in kcals. For adult women, approximately 1940 calories are

recommended per day and for men, 2550 calories. The thing is, we are all different and so this is just a starting point.

10 high-calorie foods that might surprise you (or not)

Dried apricots (20g) 240 calories

Naan bread (160g) 538 calories

Pistachio nuts (30g) 184 calories

Crème fraîche (100g) 362 calories

Chorizo (50g) 156 calories

Taramasalata (50g) 240 calories

Butter (a thin spread for a piece of toast) 51 calories

Olive oil (1 tablespoon) 127 calories

Danish pastry 411 calories

Hot chocolate 330 calories

And a few interesting alternatives

Apricot 19 calories

Half-fat crème fraîche (100g) 181 calories

Ham (50g) 57 calories

Hummus (50g) 150 calories

Fruit scone 126 calories

Tea (without milk) 0 calories

Carbohydrates

Everyone who has ever gone 'low-carb' raise their hands. The simple reason high-protein and low-carbohydrate diets are so popular is that they will help you lose weight. Fortunately, the shift in focus in recent years has been to lean protein and including a few healthy carbohydrates, but for me there is still something quite strange about diets that stop you eating fresh fruit or add huge amounts of meat into your diet to stop you feeling hungry. I'm not exactly an eco warrior, but I've read enough articles about the resources it takes to farm meat versus grow vegetables to want to make much more of an effort to add more veg into my diet.

Still, not all carbohydrates are created equal by any stretch of the imagination and there are some helpful things to know, the most significant being 'simple' versus 'complex'. Simple carbohydrates are sugars, either naturally found in foods like fruit, honey and maple syrup or refined sugars in foods like cakes, biscuits and fizzy drinks. Complex carbohydrates are starches, naturally found in whole grains, vegetables and again in some fruits, and as refined starches in foods like white bread, white pasta and cakes. Simple carbohydrates are converted into energy more quickly than complex, which is why a bowl of porridge oats will keep you going for longer in the morning than a bowl of sugary cereal. When we eat sugars in their refined state, they can often upset our blood sugar balance, causing a quick high, but sadly always followed by a deeper low – the dreaded afternoon slump. Also, when we convert food into energy too quickly, we produce too much and the excess gets stored as, you guessed it, fat. Complex carbohydrates take longer to burn and so keep us sustained throughout the day.

Complex carbs
Whole grains (oats, barley, bulgur wheat)
Bananas
Leafy vegetables
Root vegetables
Brown rice

Simple carbs
Fruit
Honey
Sugar
Sweets
Biscuits
Cakes
Pasta
Pastry
White bread

The Glycemic Index (GI)

The Glycemic Index was originally devised to help people with diabetes regulate their blood sugar levels. Then a clever so-and-so realized that whether we have diabetes or not, keeping our blood sugar on an even keel can help us calm our cravings and not overeat. Not surprisingly, unrefined grains, vegetables and beans are all low or medium on the Glycemic Index and doughnuts are very high. The sugars in fruit are generally much lower than processed sugary foods, although dates are very high (well, they are like sweets).

DOES BREAD MAKE YOU FAT?

Luzia Barclay is a herbalist I know. Luzia is also passionate about whole, healthy foods and happens to have a big herb garden at Long Crichel Organic Bakery in Dorset. So Luzia knows a thing or two about bread and has kindly explained why so many of us have a difficult digestive relationship with it.

Bread produced on an industrial scale has not been given natural time to ferment, so it needs much more yeast, extra gluten, chemical improvers and vegetable fat to produce and preserve the bread so that it stays 'fresh' on the shelf. This is called The Chorleywood Process and was created in 1961. It was also described as the 'no time' process as it sped up bread making so dramatically.

The warm, moist conditions in the digestive system are ideal for this type of bread to ferment and cause bloating in the gut. The 'worst' breads tend to be the white sliced varieties, baked on an industrial scale and containing large amounts of yeast, liquid gluten and many additives. White sliced bread hardly contains any fibre and the flour is refined, which means it raises the blood sugar levels too fast. Eating too much of it can also lead to constipation. Wholemeal bread has more fibre, but still too much gluten and yeast. In many people this can cause bloating and cramping pain in the stomach.

Sourdough bread, however, especially the wholemeal variety, has a stabilizing effect on blood sugar levels. Sourdough made traditionally uses much less yeast, a natural 'starter' and doesn't need added ingredients like vegetable fat. Its carbohydrates are slowly released and do not lead to fluctuations of blood glucose. The lactic acid bacteria and long fermentation process also prevent fermentation in one's digestive system. So you don't get hunger pangs and cravings; no bloating, no cramps.

Fibre

Carbohydrates, particularly whole grains, vegetable and fruit, also provide us with the all-important fibre in our diet, especially when we want a Flat Tummy! Soluble fibre helps guide waste products through our system and insoluble fibre acts as roughage to ease the movement of waste. But enough of that . . . here are some of the best high fibre foods:

High-fibre foods
Beans/pulses
Broccoli
Artichokes
Berries
Barley
Pears
Prunes
Avocado

Protein

Proteins help build and support our bodies, from bone repairs to feeding our immune system. Lean proteins such as fish, poultry and game are great because you get all the quality protein with less of the saturated fat, but I am still on the side of eating a little top-quality protein rather than piling up our plates. For example, look for grass-fed beef or organic chicken, because it does matter what the cows and chickens eat. If our livestock aren't eating their natural diet and nor are we, then what chance do we have? It's a bit more of a challenge for vegetarians and vegans as plant proteins aren't complete. The key is to have a balanced diet of pulses, beans, grains, vegetables, nuts, seeds, sprouts and soya.

Good protein choices
Chicken
Turkey
Poussin
Game (venison, pigeon, pheasant, guinea fowl)
Fish
Shellfish
Leafy greens
Beans and pulses
Grains

Eat in moderation
Beef
Pork
Lamb

Fats

The good news is that there are good fats, so much so that they are called 'essential'. Unfortunately we often fall for the less-good fats. Saturated fats, which are usually solid at room temperature, are thought to raise cholesterol levels if eaten in high amounts. Trans fats are mostly produced by hydrogenating (hardening) vegetable oils into solid or semi-solid fats. These have been shown to increase bad cholesterol and decrease good cholesterol. Unsaturated fats are the goodies and are essential for our brains, joints and even our hearts.

The best fats are found in their whole state, rather than being processed out of foods. So olives are, in an ideal world, better than olive oil and sesame seeds better than sesame oil. For me, at least a little olive oil is a step in the right direction. And keeping to the natural 'whole' food theme I have always preferred a small amount of butter to any amount of margarine.

Saturated fats (moderation)
Butter
Cream
Cheese
Fatty red meat
Bacon
Sausages

Trans fats (avoid)
Margarine
Some hydrogenated oils (check the label)
Often found in biscuits and mass-produced cakes

Unsaturated fats (good choices)
Olive oil
Oily fish (mackerel, sardines, salmon)
Avocados
Hazelnuts

Omega-3 and omega-6
These are essential fatty acids that we only obtain through our diet and a good balance of which promotes general health. Omega-6 fatty acids are highly prevalent in the modern diet in foods like grains and vegetable oils, while omega-3 fatty acids are less so for the majority of people, hence the reason we are encouraged to eat a portion or two of oily fish each week to create a healthy balance. Walnuts, flaxseeds and omega-3 enriched eggs are also good sources.

MUFAs

Monounsaturated (plant-based) fatty acids, or MUFAs, are fast becoming part of the diet vocabulary. They are considered to be healthy fats, particularly when it comes to heart health, and include avocados, olives, nuts, seeds and dark chocolate. There have been studies that suggest MUFAs might prevent or even target abdominal fat, but the research is still in its early days.

Water

It won't come as any surprise to read that water is key to both weight loss and our general sense of health and well-being. It nourishes our entire body, from making our skin look radiant and younger to helping our kidneys perform at their optimum. Drinking more water helps with bloating, keeps our appetite in check and, if you ever feel the start of a headache coming on, try drinking a glass of water first and see if it does the trick. But don't drink too much water with your meals, just a few sips really is all you need or a cup of herbal tea. If you drink lots of cold water at the same time as eating, you will flood your digestion, making it harder to digest and absorb the nutrients from your meal. And good digestion is essential when it comes to a flat tummy.

Alcohol

A small glass of wine at dinner will do you no harm in the flat tummy department, and a glass of red is even good for you. However, it's very easy to fall into the trap of drinking too much, too often, and for many of us, there is a clear correlation between how healthy the rest of our diet is and how much alcohol we drink. So it's not just the extra calories in that half bottle of wine, but all the nibbles that often go with it.

Salt

It's easy to assume that sea salt or rock salt is healthier than regular table salt, but chemically they are pretty much the same and the message is clear that as a nation, we simply need to eat less salt. Salt raises blood pressure and therefore increases the risk of stroke and heart disease. And from a Flat Tummy point of view, too much salt means that we are more likely to suffer from water retention. The recommended daily intake of salt shouldn't exceed 6g, but it's almost impossible to tell how much we consume if we eat processed foods. If you can cook from scratch as much as possible and eat whole foods with little or no added salt, then you will go a long way to lowering your intake of salt.

REAL FOOD

When it comes to making healthy and also delicious food choices you only really need to remember one thing, *eat real food*. In my mind, this is what the entire issue with food and our diets boils down to. If you choose real food, you not only see a big difference in your waistline, but feel like a new person too. Processed foods often contain an unnatural mix of fat, simple sugars, too many calories and not enough nutritional value. Look at the labels on foods and go for choices that use as few ingredients as possible and if you don't recognize any of the ingredients, then give them a wide berth. There, I will get off my soap box now!

Antioxidants and free radicals

The main thing for us lay people to remember is that free radicals are bad because they can cause damage to our cells, increasing the risk of disease and rate of ageing. Antioxidants help in the battle against free radicals. Berries, dark chocolate, green leafy vegetables and green tea all contain antioxidants, so eat a balanced diet with plenty of fruit and veg and you'll get your antioxidants.

Vitamins and minerals

Vitamins are organic compounds found within foods, while minerals are inorganic and so are absorbed by plants from the soil or water, hence they include compounds like iron, calcium and magnesium.

Supplements

Kelp
Luzia Barclay, herbalist, recommends kelp (bladderwrack). Kelp is a seaweed that contains many valuable nutrients. It is often used to increase the metabolic rate and digest food more efficiently. When the metabolism is slow, people put on weight easily, when it is fast, they burn the food fast. Kelp prevents the accumulation of body fat and it has a strengthening effect on the thyroid gland, the gland that regulates the metabolism.

Pro or pre biotics
Probiotics and prebiotics are both helpful for intestinal health and digestion. Probiotics contain beneficial bacteria, while prebiotics nourish the good bacteria in our gut. If

you are cleaning up your diet, then taking either of these in supplement form, and also eating plenty of natural yoghurt, will help support the changes you make and may even improve how your body absorbs nutrients. The friendly bacteria help ward off bloating and sluggishness, plus they are good for the immune system.

Milk thistle

Milk thistle is a herbal tincture nutritionists will often recommend to support your liver, so if your Flat Tummy plan includes a bit of a detox, then you might want to add milk thistle to your shopping list.

Apple cider vinegar

Apple cider vinegar has undergone a trendy renaissance recently in California. It's not exactly new though; people have used cider vinegar as a natural remedy for thousands of years and the apple cider diet became popular in the 1970s. Apparently all you need to do is take one or two teaspoons of apple cider vinegar before every meal, diluted in 250ml warm or cold water. You can add a little honey to taste. Advocates claim it reduces hunger and cravings and improves digestion. It's also said to balance glucose levels and help with candida. It's important to dilute ACV if you go the drink route as the acidity can be harmful to teeth enamel.

A good multivitamin

There are so many vitamins to choose from, but in my book it's always worth going for quality and the Solgar Multi-Nutrient is first class. It contains a list of nutri-ents as long as your arm, so if you just feel you'd like to add one supplement product to your day, then give this one a go.

Note: If you are pregnant, breastfeeding or on any medication, you always need to check with your doctor before taking any supplements.

Perfect Portions

This is helpful for when we start making changes. Just to get a sense of how much a 'portion' of foods like cereal, rice, couscous and pasta is, get out your kitchen scales this week and check. I discovered a 40g portion of muesli, which is what is often recommended on the box, looked pretty paltry in my breakfast bowls, but on the positive side, I also realized I only go for about half of the 75g that is often recommended for rice. It's all part of the essential exercise in honesty. Portions can easily creep up over time and we just get used to eating a bit too much food because it's on the plate.

And speaking of plates, swapping for smaller ones actually makes you eat less, which shows just how much our eating is psychological as well as out of physical need. I also think eating from beautiful plates is a great idea when we are being more conscious of what we're eating. I know that I savour my food more when I notice the whole presentation. The same is true for my green tea ritual. If I just dunk a tea bag in any old mug, it's alright, but if I take the time to make a lovely pot and use my Japanese cup, then it makes it just that little bit special.

With foods like risotto and pasta, it's helpful to remember that the Italians usually only have a starter portion of these foods, rather than a main. And remember that in every tablespoon of olive oil, there are over 120 calories, so while the television chefs might pour over a glug, try a drizzle.

Quick look-up guide to healthy portions

If you fear your powers of portion control have deserted you, grab a set of digital scales and see with your own eyes what a healthy portion of a particular food looks like. From a positive point of view, you will also start to notice the foods that you can have great big portions of for very few calories. I vividly remember discovering that there are only 25 calories in a whole punnet of blackberries, the equivalent of half a biscuit!

I don't distinguish between a 'losing weight' portion and a 'maintenance' portion. A healthy portion is just that – what's right for us to be our healthy weight – and for many of us, it tends to be a little less than we've become used to. I think if you try to go mad and eat minuscule portions to lose weight, then not only is it depressing while you are on your diet, but it's hard to know what to do once you reach your target weight.

Once you become familiar with what a portion looks like visually, you can then ditch the scales and use your instincts. I have a little mug I now use to measure out rice as I'm so familiar with what a portion looks like in it. When you realize how densely packed a piece of Cheddar is in terms of calories, you'll remember to cut a matchbox-size slice rather than a doorstep-size chunk.

Porridge oats 40g oats with 150ml semi-skimmed milk (rest water) with 1 tablespoon honey

Muesli 40g (look on the packet for nutrition as all are different) = 140 calories

Granola 20g is a good sprinkle = 85 calories (approx)

Couscous 40g (dry) = 148 calories

Rice
    40g (dry) long grain = 140 calories
    40g (dry) brown = 155 calories

Egg noodles 62.5g average 'nest' = 190 calories

Pasta 50g dry spaghetti = 170 calories

Vegetable oils 1 tablespoon = 120 calories

Cheese
    30g Cheddar = 123 calories
    30g cottage cheese = 30 calories
    30g Brie = 87 calories
    10g Parmesan = 40 calories
    30g feta = 90 calories

Natural yoghurt 125g pot = 120 calories

Butter 10g = 75 calories

Eggs 2 medium = 130 calories

Dark chocolate a strip is usually a 1/6 of a 100g bar = 100 calories

Hazelnuts a handful is approximately 15g = 100 calories

Jacket potato small (100g) = 136 calories

Chicken medium breast 150g = 220 calories

Salmon small 100g fillet = 200 calories

Cod 100g = 69 calories

Sea bass 100g = 140 calories

King prawns 100g = 78 calories

Tuna steak 100g = 140 calories

Tuna steak in spring water 80g (which is often about ½ a can, although they do vary) = 84 calories

Beef mince (lean) 80g = 170 calories

Pork chop (lean) 120g = 220 calories

Chipolatas 3 = 195 calories

Lamb cutlets (lean) 2 (150g) = 357 calories

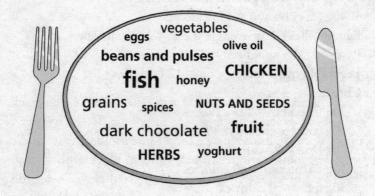

Top 20 Flat Tummy Foods

1. Green Tea

I have been lucky enough to visit Tokyo and bring back packets of green tea so vibrant in colour that whenever I make a pot, I almost feel healthier just looking at it. There are three main varieties of tea – green, black and oolong. But then, of course, there are the myriad herbal teas you can make by simply picking a few leaves off a plant and steeping them in boiling water.

Green tea is made from unfermented leaves and is thought to contain the highest levels of antioxidants, called polyphenols. These antioxidants help to neutralize, and even prevent, some of the damage cause by free radicals, little nasties that contribute to the ageing process and various health problems. Green tea is mildly diuretic, so helps the body get rid of excess water, helps with gas, is a stimulant and also helps to regulate body temperature. So if you find a cup of coffee tends to make you feel a bit hot and bothered, then try swapping to green tea for a more balanced cuppa. Green tea may help to lower overall cholesterol, raise good HDL cholesterol and has also been shown to help regulate blood sugar, which can in turn reduce sweet cravings.

Put your feet up and enjoy a lovely cup of green tea with a square of super dark chocolate!

Green tea frappé

Make a pot of fresh green tea and let it cool. Add to a blender along with a couple of handfuls of frozen mixed berries. Squeeze a bit of peeled fresh ginger through a crusher, add a good squeeze of lemon juice and a couple of ice cubes and blend for a super healthy smoothie.

2. Olive Oil

Olive trees are thought to have first been cultivated in the Middle East and Crete as long ago as 3000 BC. In these times, olive oil was not only used for cooking, but also for the body and hair, and even in the making and fuelling of lamps. My sister puts just a little olive oil in her hair to calm the frizz and add moisture; it works a treat. Olive trees adore the climate of the Mediterranean and California and it's no coincidence that the traditional Mediterranean diet is one of the healthiest in the world. Tomatoes, garlic and olive oil are at the foundation and all three are natural healers.

Olive oil is a monounsaturated fat, or MUFA as they are now often called. MUFAs are the good fats in the family and can help you maintain a lower weight. This is good news if you tend to yo yo in your weight, going up and down on the scales. By steering clear of saturated and trans fats (see page 50) and replacing these with monounsaturated fats like olive oil and avocado, you will be helping to keep your weight balanced.

The trick is to remember that olive oil is still a very rich food; yes it's good for us, but it should still be savoured in small amounts. Extra-virgin olive oil is best used to add flavour in its pure state, rather than in the cooking process as it breaks down at high temperatures. Regular olive oil can be used in cooking, but in more gentle ways like marinating meat or fish, not in the heat of a stir-fry. See page 288 where olive oil is used to cook the tomatoes for a Roasted Tomato and Basil Soup.

3. Lemon

My great grandmother swore by PLJ first thing in the morning – Pure Lemon Juice. She said it 'got her going' and that is exactly what research tells us lemon juice does, it gets our digestion going. Good digestion is essential to healthy weight loss, and it also helps prevent us feeling bloated or sluggish. When our digestion is on great form, we tend to want to feed it the right foods, another of those positive cycles. Likewise, when our digestion is struggling to get all the good nutrients out of the food we eat, it tends to send hunger signals to the brain even though we've eaten plenty.

Pectin, found in lemon peel, is a good source of fibre that helps you to feel satisfied after a meal and keep your blood sugar in a nice balance. Think where you can add lemon juice, zest or peel to your meals because it's a very handy and healthy ingredient to have around.

4. Chicken

Chicken is the natural representative for lean proteins. As I have so much respect for vegetarians and am a true believer in the side of science that advocates more vegetables in our diet, I aim for a balance. And while it might be considered a bit pale and uninteresting by some, if I could choose only one meat, then it would be the humble chicken. When I asked Flat Tummy Club members for their favourite soup recipes, chicken easily topped the list, and I know a wonderful acupuncturist and author who specializes in women's health, Emma Cannon, who could literally write a whole book on the history and benefits of chicken soup. A friend's mum contributed some delicious recipes to this very book and one of the simplest is one of the very best: chicken thighs marinated in lemon juice, zest and herbs and roasted – mouthwatering (see Lemon and Herb Chicken, page 325).

From a nutrition perspective, as a white meat, chicken has the benefits of protein without all the saturated fat of red meat. Protein is helpful for keeping you fuller for longer, but if you can keep it lean, then all the better. Chicken also contains energy-giving B vitamins. Personally, I don't like to think of chickens in cages or squashed up tight in barns, so I do look for free-range and organic and because I prefer thighs to breast, they are good value, even when organic. A tip about buying eggs is that if you can find local free-range or organic eggs, either in the farm shop or direct, then they are usually cheaper than regular supermarket eggs and have those glorious orange yolks.

5. Cinnamon

A sweet tasting spice, cinnamon is warming and stimulating for the digestion – in fact, interestingly, it stimulates and heals at the same time. Cinnamon is the dried bark of the laurel tree and has been used medicinally for over 5000 years – early Chinese texts describe using cinnamon for colds, flu and digestive disturbance. Cinnamon has been show to be particularly good for keeping your blood sugar in balance, essential when trying to lose weight.

Cinnamon is a lovely spice for adding to mild, spicy stews and also has a wonderful sweetness that goes so well with baked fruit. If you love milky lattes, then you might enjoy swapping these for a cup of chai, which I like black, but you can make with half water and half hot milk.

Green chai tea
To make a pot
1 tablespoon green tea leaves
¼ teaspoon ground ginger
3 cloves
¼ teaspoon ground cinnamon
¼ teaspoon 5-spice powder

6. Cucumber

I always thought it was just a myth that cucumber is a weight loss food, a bit like cabbage soup, and that really all vegetables are good for you. While it's true that you can't beat a rich variety of vegetables in your diet, cucumber is worth pointing out as one of those foods that is described as 'diuretic,' in that it helps the body to get rid of excess water. This is good to know when your tummy feels like a tightened drum. Just as the phrase suggests, cucumber is a cooling food, which is why we are so drawn to them in the summer and less so in the colder winter months. It's no surprise the cucumber is in the same family as the watermelon, which is also very good if you are feeling bloated or sluggish. They are naturally hydrating and the skin of a cucumber is full of fibre. I find supermarket cucumber skin gives me indigestion unfortunately, but have discovered that farm shop varieties like English Hothouse are much easier to digest. Cucumbers have long been used for their skin healing properties too, both from the inside out and from the outside in, so for glowing skin, have a cucumber salad and keep a few slices for your dark circles. See page 289 for Hot Cucumber Soup.

7. Oats

The humble oat. If one week I splurge on buying a posh granola, the next week I always feel happy to return to a simple and incredibly inexpensive bag of oats. Whether you like your porridge with a splash of milk, made like something you can build walls with or nice and soft, porridge in the morning is simply the best way to start the day. Oats are complex, as in good, carbohydrates, which release their energy slowly and steadily rather than creating a big spike from something sugary. They also ease us gently into the day as oats contain calming nutrients, help out in the fibre department and are nourishing for our tummies as they are easy to digest, especially if you soak them overnight.

When I rediscovered porridge as an adult, I tried all different types, from super deluxe organic jumbo oats to supermarket own brands. For me, the own brands win hands down because I find the slightly finer oats much easier to digest and frankly more enjoyable to eat. So if you think you don't like porridge, shop around and never be afraid to go for the simplest option. While I was losing weight, I ate porridge every day, either with a drizzle of honey or some home-made compote. My dad adds all sorts of things, from flax seeds to nuts and dried fruit. Go for it – a good breakfast really does set you up for the day and sends you off with your willpower strong and your tummy happy.

Porridge toppings

- A drizzle of honey – be sparing as honey has a lovely depth of flavour that I find you only need a little of with porridge
- Quick-and-Easy Berry Compote (see page 264)
- A spoonful of natural yoghurt and a few berries (the yoghurt is additional protein that will give you a real feeling of satisfaction if you like a BIG breakfast)
- Add a sprinkle of cinnamon, cardamom, ginger and raisins or dried cranberries as you make the porridge to give a warm and spicy flavour, lovely in the colder months
- Prunes softened in apple juice

8. Natural Yoghurt

Yoghurt is just an all round goody two shoes. It's the perfect satisfying snack if you need something mid-morning or afternoon as it's a good source of protein; the perfect afters with a little drizzle of honey; and the perfect breakfast with warm compote and a sprinkle of granola. Yoghurt is a great source of calcium and for our flat tummies it contains

Lactobacillus, those helpful bacteria that feed our intestines and improve how our digestive system absorbs nutrients. Yoghurt is also good for helping to balance yeast in the body.

Always buy plain live yoghurt and add fruit or honey to the yoghurt just before you eat it for the full effect. Check the ingredients list before buying low-fat varieties as they will often contain ingredients other than 'milk'. Natural really is best when it comes to yoghurt.

A few yoghurt tips

- For a summer treat, add a little cream to yoghurt, mix together and serve over fresh strawberries
- Squeeze lemon juice and fresh ginger into yoghurt and drizzle with honey
- If you are swapping cream for yoghurt in a recipe, add the yoghurt at the last minute and off the heat to stop it splitting

9. Beans

Now anyone who knows me will be exclaiming here, 'Beans, but Kate, you can't stand beans.' It's true, on my Flat Tummy Club culinary adventures, I have had my eyes opened to both the flavour and the healthiness of beans. On one particular occasion, I was staying with a friend for a couple of nights and while she put her children to bed, I offered to follow the vegetarian chilli recipe she had found in a magazine for our supper. I read through all the ingredients and felt a wave of apprehension – look at all those beans. Still, I got chopping and grinding and soon the chilli was bubbling away, smelling rather delicious. An hour later my friend flopped down with a bowl of steaming chilli and sour cream and soon went back for seconds. And what did I think of all those flageolet and borlotti beans? They were absolutely delicious. And I can say this because this is the Flat Tummy Club, but they also had a rather brilliant effect on my digestion, which had been ever so slightly disgruntled for a few days.

So why have I put 'beans' on the list, apart from the fact that I now like them? Well, beans really are very good for our digestion. They contain the highest levels of fibre, including both soluble and insoluble, of all vegetables (although technically beans, pulses and legumes are in a food group of their own). So in the battle to banish the bloat, you can enlist the help of beans rather than go for an expensive colonic (see page 227). Beans are also a great low-fat vegetarian source of protein, so think about swapping chilli con carne for chilli *sin* carne.

10. Turmeric

I properly discovered turmeric when I published a rather amazing book, *Anticancer* by Dr David Servan-Schreiber. *Anticancer* is in many ways a prescription for health because the anticancer food plate focuses very much on fresh vegetables, fruits, pulses and beans with a little fat, a decent, but by no means massive, portion of cereals and equal again of protein. I remember having lunch with David and he turned conventional ordering wisdom on its head by ordering a starter-size fish dish with about four separate vegetable dishes. We all followed suit and ate the most delicious and healthful meal I'd ever had in that restaurant.

Herbs and spices not only give our food a wonderful variety of flavours, but they are also packed with health and, like cinnamon, turmeric is a bit of a star. Turmeric is the most powerful natural anti-inflammatory experts know of and as well as containing anticancer properties, there is now early research that suggests it may help prevent weight gain. For the body to better absorb turmeric, mix with a little ground black pepper and dissolve in olive oil before cooking.

11. Quinoa

Quinoa (pronounced keen-wah) looks like a grain, but is actually a Peruvian seed that is related to leafy green vegetables. It contains all the essential amino acids, is high in iron and is another great protein option that is as versatile as rice. You can literally cook it in water or stock and try as an alternative to rice. And if you get bored of porridge coming out of your ears for breakfast, you can make a lovely sweet quinoa porridge with cinnamon, honey and stewed apples.

12. Pears

I remember a diet that was based on eating up to five apples a day! I'm not quite sure what that would do to my tummy, but I suspect it might put me off apples for life. Apples are fantastic, but I thought I'd redress the balance and spread the word on the humble pear. Pears are often recommended as a baby's first fruit and even as grown-ups, pears are advised for people to try if other fruit doesn't agree with them.

13. Dark Chocolate

It makes me so happy that dark chocolate is good for us. Yes, in moderation, but I don't mind, just a couple of squares with a cup of green tea and I'm set for the rest of the afternoon, with a burst of antioxidants from the chocolate and the tea. Chocolate has itself been used as a drink for around 3000 years, originating in South America. It was a bitter drink, *chocolatl,* often flavoured with vanilla and chilli. It wasn't until the Spanish conquest of the Aztecs that Europeans encountered chocolate for the first time and chocolate as a solid wasn't created until the mid 1800s. Cortez described *chocolatl* as a divine drink, which 'builds up resistance and fights fatigue'.

Many dark chocolate bars are now divided into handy squares, a strip of which add up to around 100 calories. Always look for at least 70 per cent cocoa for more health benefits and less sugar. You can melt it to add a lovely dark drizzle to baked pears or peaches, crumble it up and add to sliced banana and natural yoghurt or just enjoy as it is.

14. Berries

I will be honest here. I can't help but notice when an unfamiliar food from a far distant range of mountains turns up in our supermarkets as the new wonder superfood. Yes, I've bought my fair share of goji berries (and left them to become even more wrinkly in my desk drawer) and wondered how to pronounce 'acai'. If you happen to like a 'superfood', then great, go for it. But when I talk about berries, I mean our own native varieties, the ones we can grow and pick ourselves. In my mind they are just as super, and perhaps even more so, as tasting the sweetness of a blackberry while out for a walk in late summer and early autumn is about as good as it gets. And then I discovered that an entire punnet of blackberries is about 25 calories – that's just absurd and wonderful news. Also, snacking on berries doesn't produce a blood sugar hike and freezing berries doesn't affect their healthiness at all, so you can make your own berry compote all year round to enjoy on your morning porridge or warm up and pour over natural yoghurt for a guilt-free dessert.

15. Leeks

In France, leek soup is the slightly more appetizing equivalent of cabbage soup, used as a quick weight loss detox because leeks are a mild diuretic, or more realistically because you are bound to lose weight if you eat only leek soup for two days. However, I am a big fan of leeks in a slightly more balanced way, especially when they are super fresh and literally standing to attention, with that gorgeous colour and mild but delicious flavour. Leeks, like onions and garlic, are part of the allium family, a healthy group of vegetables that are very good for heart health and our immune systems. They are also a great vegetable for making up your five a day with ease. Add a leek to any stew you are cooking and they will also work well in many soups, though personally I would add a few other vegetables too as I don't fancy sipping leek broth all day.

16. Salmon

Whatever oily fish takes your fancy is fine by me. I've included salmon in the list because it is so easy to cook with and works with such a variety of flavours. It takes the same time to smear a salmon fillet with a bit of crushed ginger, squeeze over some lemon juice and grill as it takes to heat up a ready meal. A friend encouraged me to try poaching salmon and it's delicious, as is marinating salmon and a few veggies in a quick concoction of Asian storecupboard ingredients and stir-frying in just a few minutes.

While low in unhealthy saturated fats, the omega-3 fatty acids in fish like salmon, trout, mackerel, tuna and sardines are very good for us, even boosting our memory so fish really is brain food. Salmon is also high in protein and therefore makes you feel satisfied. A couple of meals a week featuring your favourite fish is perfect, both while losing weight and simply staying healthy.

17. Miso

Miso soup is one of the most convenient health foods you can find. All you have to do is tear open the sachet and add hot water. But what exactly is miso and what's so great about it? Miso is a Japanese seasoning of fermented soya beans and barley or rice malt, which produce a paste. Foods that are traditionally fermented contain active cultures that, like natural yoghurt, are very helpful for our digestion. It is salty so when you use it don't add any more salt to your cooking.

18. Mushrooms

Mushrooms, or fungi, are a food category all of their own, and all the varieties that you can't pronounce are particularly healthy. From a weight loss point of view, mushrooms are very low in calories and high in water content, so they are perfect for adding flavour and nutrients. Mushrooms are also an anticancer food as they stimulate the immune system. In Chinese medicine, they've been used for thousands of years to help beat off colds and flu for the same reason. There are an unbelievable 14,000 types of mushrooms,

3000 of which are edible, but you'll still never catch me foraging for mushrooms in the woods without a top mushroom-hunting professional.

You can even grow your own shiitake or oyster mushrooms on a log in your garden or on your windowsill (see Resources), which when you see the price of these more exotic mushrooms in the supermarkets, is a fantastic way to save a bit of money and have a living edible sculpture on your windowsill at the same time.

If you find the more common cultivated mushrooms like button, portobello and crimini difficult to digest, you might want to try shiitake, enoki, oyster, maitake and the like, as these seem to be easier on the digestion. My favourite way to eat mushrooms is the simplest – sautéed in a little butter on a slice of seeded or nutty toast (walnut please). They are also delicious with white fish, popped into any kind of stew and in a quick and easy omelette.

19. Eggs

Not the most glamorous of foods, but the humble egg is a firm Flat Tummy friend for those of us who like them; they are so versatile and easy. Eggs are a natural source of quality protein, B vitamins and vitamin D. My tip is to always buy your eggs locally, either organic or free-range if you can, because you will be rewarded with those deep orange yolks that happy chickens seem to produce. A woman in my mother's yoga class even takes in rescue chickens, ex-battery farm. She gently nurtures them back to full feather and, hey presto, they start laying the most wonderful eggs. When I was little and we went for Sunday walks with a picnic in the rucksack, we always had hard-boiled eggs as they are so sustaining. I am also devoted to omelettes, especially if I get home late, scrambled eggs and mush-rooms for weekend brunch and, if I'm feeling under the weather, often all I want is a soft-boiled egg and soldiers.

20. Greens

OK, it's not a huge surprise that if you eat your greens you'll be healthy and lean. Just chopping up a really fresh bunch of chard, kale, spinach or cavolo nero makes you feel healthy and you only need to take one look at these intensely coloured veg to know they are about as far away from a chip as you can get. The trick with greens is to find the varieties you really like; I'm not so thrilled with spinach, but will devour purple sprouting broccoli. Meanwhile, my mum pushes broccoli around on the plate, but can eat mounds of perfectly *al dente* spring cabbage.

Sugar Busting

You know the dreaded cycle: either you don't eat breakfast or leave it so long between meals that your body starts to crave a quick fix and looks longingly at cakes and biscuits. Or you've always had sugary drinks and can't face life without a teaspoon or three in your tea, especially when you're feeling stressed. Or you've developed a biscuit habit every time you make a hot drink – it's the only way to get through the afternoon office slump.

There are so many ways sugar creeps into our diet and our habits. And not to play it down, but I wonder if it's the thought that we will somehow lose the comfort factor or won't be able to function without sugar that is more persuasive than the reality. And not to play it up, but like any craving, you've got to really want to break the sugar habit or you'll be fighting a losing battle. Many scientists have pondered the line between sugar compulsion and addiction for decades and it's still a grey area.

The Sugar Debate

Why is sugar getting such a bad name in our fight against fat? Isn't it simply 'vital energy' or a 'prime source of life' as one Harley Street doctor described it in the 1950s? After all, we hear the term 'blood sugar' so it must be something we need?

The trouble with sugar today is that it is so refined and so prevalent in many foods that our blood sugar is often out of balance, either peaking on the high of an iced bun or descending to a sharp low just minutes later, sending messages to our brain for 'more please'. Sugar is energy dense, which might be handy if you are half way up Everest, but for most of us who work in fairly sedentary jobs, we just don't need such a concentration of energy in one hit. Over time, our body will set up its own defence mechanisms to stop sugar causing such surges in our natural blood sugar, but once we are addicted to the high, we just eat more sweet things to create the same effect.

There is still a debate over whether sugar is actually linked to obesity, but this is where I say let your common-sense rule. On my sister's birthday, we went out for a Dorset cream tea and decided to share it and just have one scone each. We didn't exactly skimp on the jam (or cream) and even after just one half, we both had major head rushes. About half an hour later, we slumped and needed a good strong cup of tea to feel human again. Now we've both broken our sugar cravings, we could feel just what it was doing to us. A couple of years ago, we wouldn't have noticed and my sister would have demanded at least two scones on her birthday.

To make the white granulated sugar we are all familiar with (was that a sharp intake of breath as all the bakers prepare themselves for this chapter) raw cane juice undergoes a great deal of processing to remove 'impurities' and leave those pure white crystals. The sugar cane is pressed and the resulting liquid is mixed with lime. It is then reduced and the liquid evaporated to leave raw sugar crystals. With most white sugar, the raw sugar is then processed again to remove the outer brown layer, phosphoric acid and calcium hydroxide or carbon dioxide are used to remove more impurities, then the sugar is filtered to remove the final traces of molasses and voilà, your white sugar is ready. Bizarrely, to make brown sugar at the end of all this processing, a little molasses is added back in. Demerara and muscovado sugars are made in earlier stages, the darker they are, the less refined. And molasses is a natural by-product of the sugar making process, the darkest of which is called blackstrap molasses.

Lightening Your Sugar Load

So you might think sugar is comforting, but it's difficult to find too many good reasons for putting it into your body. The first step in beating sugar cravings is to think about what too much sugar can do to your body.

- May contribute to PMS symptoms
- May contribute to symptoms of candida
- May contribute to symptoms of chronic fatigue
- May contribute to symptoms of anxiety and irritability
- Increases the risk of tooth decay
- May increase risk factors for heart disease

Once you are convinced you want to give sugar the heave-ho, here are some tips to help you through the day:

- It's essential to eat plenty of foods throughout the day that keep your blood sugar levels balanced. Stick with lean proteins, whole grains like oats and foods rich in good fats like fish and avocados.
- Don't go hungry and drink plenty of water and herbal teas during the day, especially green tea.
- Steer clear of processed foods as they often contain a lot more sugar than you realize. Take a good look at your breakfast cereals and things like low-fat or fat-free yoghurts, which often contain added sugar.
- If you need some sweetness in your life, then replace sugar with just a little honey or agave syrup and cut down on one major culprit at a time.
- Shake up your routine. I work at home and so I'm within arm's reach of the biscuit tin all day long. When I spent a week working in my family's gallery, upstairs in their office, I was doing the same work, but in a different location and my biscuit habit went by the wayside.
- Exercise can help because it produces a natural 'high' to replace the artificial highs you get from sugar. And with exercise you don't come crashing down once the sugar wears off.
- Be prepared for times of stress (see page 179). All our bad habits raise their ugly heads when times are tough. I don't think it's worth feeling guilty about this, but I must admit the healthier your diet in stressful times, the better you tend to cope.
- Keep busy. Boredom is sugar's best friend. Remember those children and the marshmallows (see page 38).

TEASPOONS OF SUGAR IN COMMON DRINKS

250ml Ribena = 6 teaspoons

500ml Coca Cola = 12.6 teaspoons

500ml This Water Oranges and Lemons =
  9.3 teaspoons

500ml Volvic Touch of Fruit Strawberry =
  5.7 teaspoons

500ml V Water Detox = 2.3 teaspoons

100ml Flora Pro-Activ Yoghurt Drink Strawberry =
  1.4 teaspoons

440ml Mars Refuel Sports = 14.4 teaspoons

100ml Muller Vitality Yoghurt Drink Raspberry =
  2.5 teaspoons

Source: *Daily Mail*

How about the Alternatives?

On finding out more about how sugar is made, I realized just what a natural wonder **honey** is. Our honey bees are vital to agriculture and the life cycle of so many plants, happily transporting pollen among plants and, at the same time, producing this rather amazing by-product, honey. The honeycomb is a thing of absolute geometrical precision and beauty, and I didn't know this, but honey can keep literally forever.

But does honey have the same effect on our bodies? In studies, honey has been shown to have less of an effect on the blood sugar levels of people with type 2 diabetes. However, it's good to remember that honey is actually sweeter than sugar, so the mantra of 'just a little' stays true. After all, it takes the honeybees an enormous amount of work to make just one pot of honey, so savour it and make it last!

Pure maple syrup contains fewer calories than honey and even has a few vitamins and minerals, including zinc for your immune system. So perhaps try lemon and maple syrup in hot water next time you feel a cold coming.

Agave syrup, a cactus nectar, has gained in popularity over the past couple of years as the sweet saviour. Agave ranks lower than sugar on the Glycemic Index, which rates foods on how quickly the sugars they contain get into your body. Agave also tastes much sweeter than sugar and so, like honey, a little goes much further.

I'm not keen personally on swapping sugar for **artificial sweeteners** like those found in diet colas, some yoghurts and sugar-free chewing gum, as I prefer natural foods and drinks wherever possible. Artificial sweeteners have also been shown to possibly hinder weight loss. Apparently, the sweet taste, even though artificial, makes you crave more food. So while the diet soda may contain zero calories and zero sugar, it might make you want to grab something to eat that you don't need.

There are many whole foods that are naturally sweet and as humans we are born with a tendency to seek out sweet foods because they tend to be the more ripe foods that won't poison us! I cut out processed sugar when losing weight, but I didn't go cold turkey with **fruit** and I had a drizzle of honey or agave on my morning porridge. To be honest, I think it helped a great deal as I could focus on making lasting changes to my eating habits rather than climbing the walls. I still lost

7lb in seven days and I even ate bananas, often shunned on weight loss plans!

Tales from the Club

A friend of mine who is very slim has always had a bit of a potbelly and she'd love to banish it for good. She's really very good as she runs, goes to the gym and looks fantastic. The gym has told her she's been lucky so far in that she eats pretty much anything she likes and stays slim, but as she gets older, it will start to gather a bit more around her middle. The thing is my friend has known this for about 10 years. She is a sugar addict and knows there is no magic alternative to weaning herself off the sugary teas, fizzy drinks and sweets. The key for her has been to tackle her sugar challenge when she's not so stressed or busy at work – when she's in a good frame of mind. That way she will break the cycle for when times next get stressful . . . so far, it's been so good.

3

GET SET . . .

About You

How is your food diary looking? Now that we have done lots of preparation thinking, building up our resolve and our knowledge, it's the perfect time to set our intention goals and our plan for how to get there.

The next step is to fill in a bit more detail about you. A good time to do this is first thing in the morning and then when you weigh yourself weekly, do so at the same time each week. I also took a few measurements with a tape measure and even now I'm surprised at the difference I discovered months later – my thighs in particular!

Weight: ....

Chest: ....

Waist (most narrow bit): ....

Tummy (widest bit): ....

Hips: ....

Thigh (just one!): ....

BMI

Most of us are very familiar now with the Body Mass Index, and although there is no 100 per cent foolproof way to discover your perfect weight, the BMI chart is helpful because it does include a healthy range.

		Height														
	Cm	150	152.5	155	157.5	160	162.5	165	167.5	170	172.5	175	177.5	180	182.5	185
	Feet	5'0"	5'1"	5'2"	5'3"	5'4"	5'5"	5'6"	5'7"	5'8"	5'9"	5'10"	5'11"	6'0"	6'1"	6'2"
Lb	Kg															
100	45	20	19	18	18	17	17	16	16	15	15	14	14	14	13	13
105	47	21	20	19	19	18	17	17	16	16	16	15	15	14	14	13
110	50	21	21	20	19	19	18	18	17	17	16	16	15	15	15	14
115	52	22	22	21	20	20	19	19	18	17	17	17	16	16	15	15
120	54	23	23	22	21	21	20	19	19	18	18	17	17	16	16	15
125	57	24	24	23	22	21	21	20	20	19	18	18	17	17	16	16
130	59	25	25	24	23	22	22	21	20	20	19	19	18	18	17	17
135	61	26	26	25	24	23	22	22	21	21	20	19	19	18	18	17
140	63	27	26	26	25	24	23	23	22	21	21	20	20	19	18	18
145	66	28	27	27	26	25	24	23	23	22	21	21	20	20	19	19
150	68	29	28	27	27	26	25	24	23	23	22	22	21	20	20	19
155	70	30	29	28	27	27	26	25	24	24	23	22	22	21	20	20
160	72	31	30	29	28	27	27	26	25	24	24	23	22	22	21	21
165	75	32	31	30	29	28	27	27	26	25	24	24	23	22	22	21
170	77	33	32	31	30	29	28	27	27	26	25	24	24	23	22	22
175	79	34	33	32	31	30	29	28	27	27	26	25	24	24	23	22
180	82	35	34	33	32	31	30	29	28	27	27	26	25	24	24	23
185	84	36	35	34	33	32	31	30	29	28	27	27	26	25	24	24
190	86	37	36	35	34	33	32	31	30	29	28	27	26	26	25	24
195	88	38	37	36	35	33	32	31	31	30	29	28	27	26	26	25
200	91	39	38	37	35	34	33	32	31	30	30	29	28	27	26	26
205	93	40	39	37	36	35	34	33	32	31	30	29	29	28	27	26
210	95	41	40	38	37	36	35	34	33	32	31	30	29	28	28	27
215	98	42	41	39	38	37	36	35	34	33	32	31	30	29	28	28
220	100	43	42	40	39	38	37	36	34	33	32	32	31	30	29	28
225	102	44	43	41	40	39	37	36	35	34	33	32	31	31	30	29
230	104	45	43	42	41	39	38	37	36	35	34	33	32	31	30	30
235	107	46	44	43	42	40	39	38	37	36	35	34	33	32	31	30
240	109	47	45	44	43	41	40	39	38	36	35	34	33	33	32	31
245	111	48	46	45	43	42	41	40	38	37	36	35	34	33	32	31
250	114	49	47	46	44	43	42	40	39	38	37	36	35	34	33	32

Weight

Weight in pounds x 704 ÷ (height in inches)^2:
. . . .

Your BMI = ...

Underweight: below 18.5
Normal: 18.5–24.9
Overweight: 25–29.9
Obese: over 30

I am 5'2" and I weighed 11 stone so my BMI was:

$$11 \times 14 \times 704 \div (5 \times 12 + 2)^2 = 28.2$$

Clearly overweight and heading towards obese. To get back into the ideal range I needed to weigh less than 9½ stone, so I set that as my initial target. Once I reached that, I kept going into the middle of ideal and a BMI of 22.

Your goal weight = ...

Waist to Hip Ratio

This is a useful formula for checking if you are more of an apple than a pear and tend to store extra weight around your tummy. Pear-shaped people are lucky in that a bit of extra weight on the bum and thighs doesn't carry the same extra health risks as weight around the abdomen. The more dangerous fat is called 'visceral' and is stored behind the abdomen wall. This is associated with an increased risk of cancer and stroke. The less dangerous fat is 'subcutaneous'. This is the kind you can pinch and is usually stored in that lower part of the tummy rather than up around the waist, as well as in the hips and thighs.

Apparently where we tend to store fat has a great deal to do with our genetics, but the good news is that visceral fat is a bit easier to budge than subcutaneous, especially with exercise.

For women

Divide your waist measurement by your hip measurement. Ideally this number should be less than 0.8.

For men

Ideally when you divide your waist measurement by your hip measurement, the figure you come up with should be less than 0.95.

Before

Ask a friend or loved one to take photos of you today – front, side and back. My friend and I squeezed into our old jeans and had a right laugh. You could also find a really good picture to inspire you or hang on for your 'after shot'.

Setting Your Goals

The key to setting any goals in life is to be specific, realistic and don't just come up with the end goal, but also how and when you will achieve it. The goal of 'losing weight' has been shown to be a bit rubbish when it comes to likely success – it's just too vague and doesn't have any actions associated with it.

Specific goal = Lose 20 pounds to reach 9 stone in 6 months, by really going for it in the first 3 weeks and by making genuine changes to my lifestyle that I embrace and will last.

It's the same for anything in life. We might have a vague goal to change our job, but the reality is that we'll never do it until we sit down and add specific detail, both to the goal itself and how we're going to make it happen. Yes, it's a form of positive thinking, but instead of relying on the universe to somehow answer our prayers, we realize it's really up to us.

For me, the goal of 'losing weight' didn't have much meaning to it. I really wanted to *feel* better in my body – more energetic, more confident. When I attached these meanings to the goal, I became so much more focused on making it happen.

Your specific goal = ...

....

Setting Your Time Frame

It's important to be aware of timing, both in the short and the long term. The first obvious, but essential, step is to choose your start week carefully. If you are incredibly busy at work or at home with little ones, then you might make a vague promise to start the plan and then find out that you're just not really up for it. For everyone, whether you have a long-term game plan to lose a significant amount of weight or you want to get in shape for your holiday in a month's time, the absolute key is to gear yourself up mentally and practically and *go for it* in the first week. We've been through the mental preparation and in the next chapters I've included all the practical preparation you need.

If you start with a fully committed week, you can expect to lose anything up to 7lb, which I did, although everyone is different. We can lose up to about 4lb of body fat in a week and any more than that will be excess water. After the euphoria of the first week, the speed of weight loss will slow down, but I know from experience it's a mental tonic to have such a strong start. It took me four weeks to lose another half stone, so aim to lose between 1-2lb on average each week. But I'm not keen on trying to work to a grid or a graph, for most of us women our hormones can affect our weight by a good few pounds for a week of every month. Keep mindful of the big picture as you start each week: make notes on how you are doing, your weight, what went well in the previous week, what you're aiming to achieve this week and remind yourself, it's definitely all worth it!

Your time frame =...

Now you have set your intentions, written down your goals and time frame, the next section is a questionnaire that will help you to identify the specific practical actions you are going to make.

The Flat Tummy Club Inquisition

Pull out your diary and keep it handy as you go through the following questionnaire. I'm sure you have already spotted the key changes that you'd need to make to reach your Flat Tummy goals and perhaps there are things that are hiding, but will come out in the open as you go through the questions. Also, identify all the healthy things you do and eat or drink already, as often it's a case of upping the ante with what you already like and enjoy. The purpose of the questionnaire is to then identify up to six changes that will form the foundation of your very own, very personal Flat Tummy Club plan.

Whenever I answer a questionnaire, I always make myself out to be a bit healthier than I truly am, even though the only person who will ever see the results is me. Be honest with yourself and take a second look.

Make a note of your answers to help analyze your habits.

Questions

DIET

1. How many cups of regular tea and/or cups/shots of regular coffee do you drink on average per day?

2. How many caffeinated (including sugar-free) or sugary soft drinks do you drink on average per day?

3. How many glasses of wine/pints of beer/shots do you drink on average per week?

4. How many glasses of water and cups of herbal tea do you drink on average per day?

5. How many teaspoons of sugar do you add to your food or drinks on average per day?

6. When you have a hot drink, do you tend to reach for an accompanying biscuit?

7. Do you regularly add salt to your cooking and food?

8. Put this list of snacks in order of your heart's desire!

   a) crisps
   b) Dairy Milk chocolate bar
   c) fruit
   d) biscuits
   e) carrot sticks and houmous
   f) sweets
   g) miso soup

9. Do you have white potatoes with most meals?

10. Do you ever eat ready meals?

11. Do you get your 5 fruit and veg portions every day?

    a) always
    b) most days
    c) not very often

12. How many portions of fish do you eat on average per week?

13. What is your typical lunch?

14. What are your nemesis foods/drinks that you suspect are not helping with the battle of the bulge?

    a) sweets (not of the fruit persuasion)
    b) sugar
    c) chocolate
    d) cakes/treats
    e) biscuits
    f) hot chocolate
    g) milky drinks
    h) cheese
    i) crisps
    j) bread
    k) potatoes
    l) pastry
    m) pasta
    n) alcohol

LIFESTYLE

15. Do you eat breakfast every day?

16. Do you go to the loo (you know what I'm saying) at least once a day?

17. Do you love to cook?

18. In times of stress, do you turn to or away from food?

19. Do you bolt your food?

20. Do you pile up food on your plate and eat until you feel stuffed?

21. Do you take regular exercise, like a brisk 30 to 45 minutes walking, jogging, swimming, a gym visit, yoga or Pilates? How many times on average per week?

Answers

1. If you drink more than 2 cups of coffee or 4 cups of tea a day, then you need to cut down on your caffeine intake. If you want a complete fresh start, then you might consider replacing coffee and regular tea with herbal alternatives, or enjoy a cup of tea or coffee in the morning and replace your afternoon drinks. We all react in our own way to caffeine. If you know you are sensitive to the effects and feel jittery or wired after a cup of coffee, then perhaps see if you actually think more clearly without the hit. Order a regular caffe latte in most coffee shops now and you get a massive cup of hot milk with a vague flavour of coffee in return. At an average of 260 calories, these can certainly add up. Swap for a small americano or cappuccino and you'll reduce that by about 150 to 200 calories in the blink of an eye.

2. If you drink any caffeinated or sugary carbonated drinks, it's helpful to know that these are a double

whammy on your tummy as the bubbles are bloating and all that sugar goes straight to your middle. Sugar-free fizzy drinks have also been shown to make us more prone to weight gain as they tend to stimulate appetite. The good news is that there are lots of delicious alternatives to try, from ginger and lemongrass cordial to green tea and pomegranate. And for a touch of nostalgia, it's easy to make your own Lemon and Ginger Barley Water for the perfect summer refreshment (see page 231).

3. Reaching for a glass of wine or a beer at the end of most days is an easy habit to fall into. For a dramatic effect on your waistline and your quality of sleep and energy, give up alcohol for the 21 days of the plan. This was my toughest challenge, but I felt amazing after just a week and by breaking the habit of mindless drinking, I now appreciate a really good glass of wine so much more.

4. One of the absolute best ways to jump start weight loss and feel more energized is simply to drink 6 to 8 glasses of water or cups of herbal tea a day. It's a weird fact, but this way you will flush out any water retention (and so help to beat the bloat, always good). Water is also fantastically hydrating for your skin. You can use all the lotions and potions in the world, but water is the best anti-ager of them all. Don't drink lots of water with your meals though, as this doesn't help with digestion. Another good tip is to eat plenty of foods that are naturally high in water content – soups, vegetables and fruit in particular.

5. If you love sugar in your tea, then breaking the habit and swapping to herbal teas will set you firmly on the path to a Flat Tummy. I didn't like green tea all that much when I first tried it, but have since acquired a real passion for it. But I'll never acquire a passion for fruit teas, so don't be put off if you've tried chamomile and can't stand it or peppermint tea isn't for you. There's such a wide choice now I'd urge you to look beyond the big brands and try flavours like chai, nettle or Rooibos. This one change will make a big difference.

6. Reaching for a biscuit every time you have a hot drink can add anything between 200 to 500 calories to your day. I swapped biscuits for clementines when I started the plan and now go for whatever seasonal fruit is on hand. Biscuits are often something we eat without thinking, so if they're not there it's surprising how little we miss them.

7. If we consume too much salt (see page 52), then we tend to retain more water – not good for our flat tummies or our digestion. Conventional cooking wisdom might suggest that salt brings out the flavour of many foods, but you really can train your taste buds to be less reliant on salt and also get to know herbs and spices better to add your flavour punch.

8. It's obvious which are the healthy snacks in this list, but when we're in the habit of eating less healthily, we don't seem to exactly crave miso soup or carrot sticks and hummus. The good news is that there are lots of delicious healthy snacks to try (see page 119) and it's crucial to fill your cupboards and handbag/briefcase with these

both during the plan and beyond. Before my 'transformation' I never thought of myself as a carrot stick girl, but now I find them sweet and the perfect nibble early evening as I make dinner.

9. Potatoes are so versatile, but they offer little nutrition for lots of starchy carbohydrate and don't even count as a portion of your daily fruit and veg. If you're looking to lose weight, then swapping potatoes for another vegetable, grain or pulse and exploring the huge variety of choices on offer is a simple change to make and makes a big difference.

10. For the next 21 days and beyond, ban ready meals from your cupboards. You can find the odd healthy ready meal nowadays, but it's important to get back into cooking real, natural foods and leave all the various additives and extra salt behind.

11. Whatever the scientists say, when I eat lots of fruit and vegetables, I'm slimmer, I don't seem to get so many colds and I just feel better. It's taken a while to fire up a passion for these healthy foods, but learning about seasonality, wild food and getting into the infinite world of soups has been a dramatic change for me since I started my quest for a flatter tummy. Add more fruit and veg to your diet through snacks, big salads, soups and sides.

12. Fish are an excellent choice once or twice a week for their high protein and essential fats. Frozen fish fillets are a great stand-by, as are frozen prawns. Or see what looks lovely and fresh on the fish counter once a week. I also find tinned tuna and sardines very handy and

salmon, trout or mackerel pâtés make for a lovely lunch on toasted soda bread with a handful of cherry tomatoes.

13. Fortunately, the soup revolution is going strong on the high street, along with sushi and salads that feature a lot more than lettuce, cucumber and tomato. Our lunch choices can have a significant impact on our energy levels for the rest of the afternoon, so really think about how you can fit a healthy lunch into your day, whether you make it yourself or you tend to pop out from work. Think less bread and go for options that are as natural and home-made-like as possible. Another great tip for lunch is to have a gentle stroll or even just a quiet sit after your lunch before you get on with the day. Often we try to go full steam ahead into the afternoon and then need a pick-me-up an hour later, while we actually need to let our food digest a bit first.

14. We all have our 'nemesis' foods, which is what I term the foods that if they are in the kitchen cupboard, don't stay there for long and make us feel rather weak and feeble-willed. Kick these into the long grass for the next 21 days to get back your sense of control and balance.

15. A healthy breakfast of oats, yoghurt or eggs boosts your brainpower, willpower and mood, plus eating breakfast is essential if you're going to lose weight and keep it off happily. For the vast majority of people, if you don't eat breakfast then sometime around mid-morning your blood sugar will dip, sending a message to your brain along the lines of 'I need something fast

to boost my energy.' And there is nothing faster than sugar, hence the craving.

16. Going to the loo regularly and yes, I have to say it, plentifully, is good for your general health and wellbeing and also your Flat Tummy. The more fibre you eat in the form of fruit, vegetables and whole grains, the better your digestion and the better you feel.

17. A passion for healthy cooking is a shortcut to a Flat Tummy. Unfortunately 'passion' and 'healthy' don't often go together in the same sentence, but once you start to explore recipes from around the world, become a local food expert or have to use your culinary imagination every week when the veg box arrives, you will realize that cooking with nature's ingredients is about as good as it gets. Often we feel we don't have the time or energy to cook, but it's actually quite therapeutic to chop a few vegetables and whip up a stir-fry rather than stick something in the microwave.

18. No scientist has ever really explained to me why on earth so many of us seem to instinctively reach for the foods and drinks that will make our stress or tiredness worse rather than better. Dealing with your stress (see page 179) might be the one major key you need to unlock your weight loss.

19. Eating slowly and enjoying your food has been shown to help with weight loss. There are a few good reasons for this: we realize quicker that we are full; we help with digestion by introducing food to the stomach more slowly and already masticated; and enjoying food also stimulates stomach juices for a more efficient absorption of the nutrients.

20. Perfect portions (see page 55) are the best friend of Flat Tummy Club. Serving up on smaller plates has been shown to help us eat less. Watch your portions and make sure you're eating just enough rather than feeling a bit full. And girls, I've got to say this, but do you need the same amount as a bloke?

21. If you said yes then great, get planning more exercise for the week ahead. If you said no then I promise there is an exercise out there for everyone. Read Flat Tummy Exercise (see page 99) before you start your plan and gear yourself up, even if it's for a walk in the park. Exercise makes losing weight so much easier, it clears your mind and keeps your body fit as well as slim.

Your Plan

Here are a few ideas that might resonate with you for your plan. And of course, do add your own.

- Explore the world of herbal teas
- Drink more water to boost energy and add a sparkle to my eyes
- No more sugar – go for natural sweeteners like fruit and a little honey
- Ditch the mindless drinking
- Instead of salt, pack my cupboards with spices and herbs
- Be generous to myself with healthy snacks
- Find alternatives for my nemesis foods
- Swap white potatoes for other vibrant vegetables, beans and pulses

- Become a soup addict
- Less wheat and gluten
- Five fruit and veg a day
- Try a fish recipe at least once a week
- Eat a healthy breakfast
- Replace processed foods with real foods; refined grains with whole
- Cook from scratch
- Plan meals so I don't get caught out
- Fill my fridge with healthy foods I love
- Savour my food and eat slowly, being aware of my portions
- Exercise!

My friends tell me I did all of the above, so that's why I was so successful. When I look at the list I realize that yes, I planned, prepared and became a complete goody two shoes, but I didn't have to carry around a list of banned foods or start calculating my calorie intake for the day. I put my focus on the six things I knew I would struggle with:

Kate's Plan 'Little and Often'

Replace crisps, cheese, bread, white potatoes and alcohol
Healthy snacks – two every day
Good breakfast, one main meal and one lighter meal (soup or salad) a day – better planning
Drink lots of herbal tea
Lots of walking
Five fruit and veg a day

Your Plan

....

....

....

....

....

....

Flat Tummy Exercise

It's pretty obvious by now, but I am a great believer in balance when it comes to a healthy lifestyle. So even if you *think* you hate exercise, I'm not about to promise that you can lose weight, keep it off *and* feel great without doing any.

What I do know is that the gym definitely isn't for everybody, so the key is to keep exploring until you find a form of exercise you enjoy. Walking is the perfect exercise for anyone getting started and for keeping slim and healthy – find a way to fit a few hours into your week and you will reap huge benefits. And do give different things a few tries before you write them off – it took me about six workout classes before I started to look forward to Tae Bo rather than feel like it was a chore. I always felt good afterwards, but had to drag myself there, until one evening I found I wasn't trying to make up excuses in my head for not going. But it can take a while before exercise is something we instinctively want to do. Often our willpower fails us and we find ourselves not bothering to take the stairs, walk up the escalator or go to our Pilates class. Be aware of those lazy habits and keep thinking all the time of how you actually feel when you do exercise, when your body releases all those feel-good hormones, tension flows away and you feel that sense of 'good tired'.

Write down whatever exercise you manage in your food diary to see how you are getting back into the swing of it. And block off time in your calendar for exercise. If you don't think there's enough time in the day to fit in exercise, then the one most important thing that will lead to Flat Tummy success is to find that time.

One incentive is to think of the 'after burn' effect of exercise. This is where you continue to burn calories at a faster rate long after you have finished exercising – up to 24 hours. So if you exercise during the day, your body will still enjoy the benefits as you sleep. And another incentive that really works is to sign up, even better with a friend, for a charity exercise event. This might be trekking to Mount Everest Base Camp or a 5k run. If you need to train for it, then it's the perfect motivation to take you off the sofa and get moving.

Fitting More Movement into Your Day

When I started my plan, I would look for the little things I could do in my daily life that kept me moving. It was as much a psychological boost as a physical one as I felt more alert and that I was becoming generally more energetic.

- Walk up the escalators
- Take the stairs instead of the lift
- Get off a tube stop before yours and walk the rest of the way
- If you work in an office, get up from your desk every hour for a stretch of the legs (and make a cup of herbal tea)

- Pop outside at lunchtime for a walk, even for 10 minutes

Walk Yourself Slim

Yes, it's obvious, but walking is *so* good for us. Not only do you burn calories and tone up, but you get to clear your mind, perhaps explore the countryside or discover interesting routes through town and perk up your energy levels all at the same time.

I am lucky that my family have walked (and often got lost) from as far back as anyone can remember. Both my parents are Londoners, but they share a passion for nature and many of my earliest memories are being taught the names of trees while we stopped for a ham roll and a hard-boiled egg. It was actually depressing for me when I was injured and unable to walk; I didn't know what to do with myself. But then, over time, I got into the habit of not walking and even when I was all better, whole weekends would drift by without a walk, sapping my energy even more. I got lazy.

A crucial part of my turnaround was always going to be getting walking back into my life. I was military about it to start with because that's what I needed to get into the swing of it – every single night it didn't pour with rain I walked either to or from, and often both ways, to the station, about 45 minutes each way. In the evenings it was dark and wintry, but the added bonus was that I'd arrive home having let go of the day and feeling relaxed and refreshed. I walked during the time I would usually just laze about in front of the television eating snacks and drinking wine, and by the time I got through the door, I would simply wander straight into the kitchen and prepare supper. I can't pretend it was easy every single day, but once I saw the difference it made on the bathroom scales, even in a week, I discovered this was a habit I could enjoy. And according to the National Weight Control Registry in the USA (see Resources), 94 per cent of the participants (all of whom have lost weight and kept it off over time) reported that they had increased their physical activity, the most reported form of exercise being walking.

It might sound silly, but I got started by wearing a pedometer. You fill in your weight and stride length, attach the pedometer to your belt and off you go. The pedometer counts your steps, calculates the distance and even gives the approximate number of calories you have burned. You can see how many steps you take in an average day and then set some upwardly mobile goals.

Walking is even getting trendy. In my local park and all over the country, you can turn up to try Nordic Walking for extra burn (see Resources). This is where you use poles to work your upper body at the same time and also use the support of the poles to work that extra bit harder and faster. Apparently it's one of the fastest-growing activities in the world. And if you don't fancy all that pole business, then it's also a great idea just to meet up with a friend for a brisk walk. I keep noticing women doing this both here in the UK and wherever I go in the world, and it's such a good idea. Of course the first place I discovered people 'walking themselves slim' was in California. I must admit walking along the bay looking at the Golden Gate Bridge is just about the perfect incentive.

If you live in a major city, check out the site www.walkit. com. You can type in your planned walk and not only get directions, but an average step count, journey time and calories burned. If I'm going out for lunch in London, I will often look at walkit to find a walk before or afterwards that goes some of my way home. When I take the 'less busy' route, I always discover interesting back streets, shops and galleries, so get a cultural tour at the same time as burning off my lunch.

Jogging and Running

I was a good hockey player back in my school days, but my coaches despaired of me, 'If only you would run a bit more, Kate!' I will be honest, things haven't changed, but enough of my friends talk evangelically about jogging and running for me to realize that for many people it's an ideal exercise. It's especially good if you have young children, as many people I know take it in turns with their partner to go for a half-hour jog in the morning or evening. It really does blow the cobwebs away and is the type of exercise that is perfectly suited to having mini goals. A friend of mine was keen to get jogging again a few months after having her second baby. She lives on a huge hill so it's difficult to just step out the door and run with a buggy. So she rented a treadmill to see if it might do the trick and loved it, putting the music on and building up her stamina in her own time. Now she's doing the London Marathon!

Beginners' tips for jogging

- Start very gradually and work up to 30 minutes over time. Half an hour jogging, two to three times a week, is perfect.
- Warm up by doing some simple stretches for 3 to 5 minutes before you start jogging (see page 377–378 for recommended stretch routines).

- If you can only jog for a couple of minutes to start with, it doesn't matter. Alternate jogging for walking, and then jog for another couple of minutes. Keep going for 30 minutes, even if the majority of that time is spent walking to begin with.
- Warm down with a few minutes stretching at the end.
- Do invest in a good pair of running shoes. If you go to your local sports shop, they will be able to recommend what's right for you.
- Your breathing rhythm will come naturally. If you are struggling to catch your breath, always ease down and if you need to, stop and allow yourself to recover.

Cycling

I live near a big park in London that is just the right distance for me to cycle round and feel like I've had a really good workout. Cycling is excellent because it works your muscles and gets your heart rate up without putting pressure on your joints in the same way that running can. It's a brilliant Sunday afternoon family activity or a way to commute to work, and you can easily chart your progress in terms of whether the hills ever start to get any easier. I see lots of mothers cycling with their children to school near me and always think what a great way to start the day for both the mums and the kids. Of course, it's just not practical for everyone, but if you can fit cycling into your daily life, it's a fantastic way to get lots of fresh air, keep fit and burn off a few calories all at the same time.

The same piece of advice is true for buying any sports or fitness equipment – never be afraid to ask the shop assistant for their advice. For example, Evans is a brilliant chain of cycle shops and they really know their stuff. They won't suggest you buy a racing bike if you're just starting out, but also you might be better off with a road bike rather than a mountain bike, depending on where you live. And the best tip is to simply make sure you keep pedalling rather than freewheeling wherever possible (except when hurtling down the hill of course). Here's what one happy Flat Tummy Club cyclist says:

I guess it's all about finding the thing that fits in to your life without too much effort. It's cycling for me – I cycle to work at least once a week, which is 8 miles one way. Sometimes I just do one way and leave my bike at work and cycle back the next. I thought it would be impossible, but actually it's fine – I just potter along and it takes about an hour, which is still quicker than public transport and cheaper too. And because I go slow and steady, I don't bother with any special lycra clothes or have to change.

Pilates

Joseph Pilates developed this form of exercise in the early twentieth century as a therapy to help strengthen his body after suffering from asthma and rickets as a child. Interned during the First World War, Pilates helped fellow internees keep healthy and strong, and then after the war, Pilates emigrated to New York where he set up his first studio.

Pilates seems to gain in popularity year on year and it's especially good for developing lean muscles while also being very relaxing for the mind. Pilates is a slow workout – often the slower the better – and so it is for strength, rather than aerobic fitness. It all centres around 'the core', which is why it has become such a useful tool of physio-therapy, strengthening your abdomen to in turn support your back, help with balance, posture and flexibility. And of course, all that focus on the core is especially good for flat tummies.

My favourite introduction to Pilates is the book or DVD *Pilates for Life* by Darcey Bussell (see Resources). As a ballerina, Darcey did Pilates every day, but she also likes to keep things simple and the explanations of the exercises in her book are simple enough for even a beginner to follow for 10 minutes a day. There are also Pilates classes and one-to-one teaching available throughout the UK, and I always think the best thing is to go on personal recommendation.

Yoga

Yoga is a total mind-body exercise that also increases flexibility and strength. With much focus on the breath, yoga works your body while relaxing your mind. It's thousands of years old, originating in India, but is just as popular as ever so must be good because it's never gone out of fashion.

Hatha yoga

'Ha' is Sanskrit for 'sun', while 'tha' is the word for 'moon', and so the aim of Hatha yoga is for balance between body and mind. Hatha yoga classes are nearly always slow moving with a focus on the positions, breathing and usually with an element of meditation. The earliest reference to yoga can be found in the *Rig Veda*, the earliest Vedic text and one of the oldest books known to man (between 1500 and 3000 BC). So yoga has certainly stood the test of time, which I think is all the evidence needed to know it's pretty good for us.

Bikram or hot yoga

A more recent adaptation of yoga was created by Bikram Choudhury and is fast growing in popularity. It is a series of 26 yoga poses, which are done in a room heated to just over 100 degrees Fahrenheit. The heat is said to warm, and therefore soften, your body so that you can perform the poses with even more flexibility. It sounds a bit extreme for me, but whatever takes your fancy.

Swimming

Swimming is a fabulous form of exercise that puts no pressure on your joints. That said, people with certain back problems may find breaststroke is not great and so if you can, front crawl or backstroke are best.

I find that now I'm more aware of my stomach muscles through other forms of exercise, I pay more attention to these while I'm swimming, but if I'm honest, swimming is something I do on holiday rather than every week at the local indoor pool. The good thing is that now I feel more confident on the beach and by the pool, I will actually go for a swim rather than lie horizontal for as long as possible as a way of hiding.

The Gym

The last time I was a paid-up member of a gym was 15 years ago. I'm jealous of people who love the gym because you can do a workout whenever you want, whatever the weather. If you are new to the gym, beware the New Year trap when there seem to be good deals around, but what often happens is that you end up paying a big monthly fee and you hardly ever go. I would start with a gym where you can pay one month at a time or even one visit at a time. You might want to start with a series of personal training sessions to make sure you go. The only problem is that I know too many people who started out this way, but as soon as the sessions ended, they stopped going to the gym. It's easier if you have a friend with iron gym-going will-power, but if you really struggle with exercise, then do consider if you can afford to pay for a trainer once a week.

Classes

If you've tried going to a big, shiny gym and found it off-putting and intimidating, then don't worry because there are so many choices when it comes to exercising, especially in a group.

I had never done an exercise class in my life until just before writing this book, which shows it's never too late to change. A friend told me about her Monday evening Tae Bo workout class and invited me along. Tae Bo, or kickboxing, workouts are a modern keep-fit twist combining martial arts moves with aerobics, and often with an abs workout thrown into the mix. If you struggle to push yourself at the gym or out for a jog, then joining a class is a guaranteed hour of working hard and building up a sweat.

It was about as perfect a class as I could go to – round the corner from the tube in a local arts centre. There was no glamour, to be honest the rooms are a bit hot, but that meant all the pressure to look good went out the window and we could just relax and have a laugh while working up a real sweat. For some, the glamour is all part of the appeal. I remember sitting outside a coffee shop in LA, above which there was a yoga school and as I watched all the class goers arrive, I tried not to stare at their amazing outfits (even their mat bags were gorgeous). Perhaps I will advance to that stage one day, but in the meantime I'm happy my friend convinced me to go along to Tae Bo. Yes, our instructor despairs of us when we forget what he taught us just a week before and when I struggle with any move that requires a degree of rhythm or coordination, but we have an hour of fantastic exercise and even get serenaded by the Turnham Green 'Glee' club on our way out.

There are yoga, Pilates, salsa, Zumba, kickboxing, Ski Fit, Nordic Walking, kettle bells, Military Fitness and many more classes going on in community halls, school gyms and parks all over the country. And now I can say from personal experience that if you want a bit of a laugh with some lovely people you might only see once a week for an hour of jumping around, then go for it – join a class near you and give it a whirl.

Do Whatever Takes Your Fancy

Whether you can take up tennis with a friend, join the local rowing club or you think golf is more your thing, give it a go. It's easy to dismiss exercise as something we hate because it's associated with grim PE lessons at school. Why they don't include things like yoga and Pilates in schools I don't know. For many women, it's an unconscious reminder of the difficulties of puberty and not feeling comfortable with our bodies; I know I still have a 'thing' about changing rooms. But I can say, hand on heart, that finding an exercise you enjoy is worth so much in terms of wellbeing and it also means you don't have to fixate on food to lose weight or stay slim. You can be more relaxed, which in my book, is always a good thing.

Top tip

If you exercise on an empty stomach you will burn more fat, rather than burning off what you have just eaten. But you want to have the energy to work hard and Noel at Tae Bo says bananas are the best if you need a snack ahead of a workout.

> ## 30 MINUTES OF . . .
>
> **Cycling = 171 calories**
> **Golf = 150 calories**
> **Jogging = 233 calories**
> **Salsa dancing = 150 calories**
> **Skiing = 186 calories**
> **Step aerobics = 223 calories**
> **Swimming = 171 calories**
> **Tennis = 171 calories**
> **Washing the car = 100 calories**
> **Weeding = 150 calories**
> **Walking (medium pace) = 129 calories**

Healthy Kitchen

To become a cook you only need a few essentials: appetite, ingredients, a kitchen to work in, a few tools and a few ideas about what to cook. But which comes first? Appetite, perhaps: the one thing that all the people I know who love to cook have in common is that they love to eat – and the desire to eat good food is what motivated them to become good cooks.
– Alice Waters, *The Art of Simple Food*

Often diet or health food is not exactly synonymous with passion, enjoyment or, indeed, appetite. Ironically, I have become more passionate about food and ingredients since making a healthy change than before when I was too stressed to care. I only really discovered the huge array of spices and herbs that built up in my kitchen cupboard over the years when I started to think about how to add different flavours to soups, stir-fries, stews and, well, everything. I'm gradually learning more and more about eating seasonally and how nature amazingly provides certain nutrients we need and flavours we crave at different times of the year. For example, nuts are packed with minerals that help boost our mood during the dark winter months and root vegetables are naturally sweet when we need warmth and comfort during the colder seasons.

I've included a section of recipes at the end of the book, some of which I used to get my new and improved healthy lifestyle started, plus some welcome contributions from the Flat Tummy Club. You can also go to the Healthy Recipes section of the website for more ideas and please do add your own for us all to enjoy. My favourite ingredients and healthy cooking tips are listed below, but it's always a matter of personal taste, so have a look through your own cookbooks and explore your imagination.

Right now give your fridge and kitchen cupboards their own detox. As a brilliant health author I know once said to me, don't think you have to use up all the bad foods because it feels wrong to throw food away . . . why use your body as a rubbish bin? Have a good rummage and why not have a spring clean at the same time? Start afresh and burn a few calories!

Flat Tummy Shopping List

There is a fantastic book by Michael Pollen titled *In Defence of Food* that describes the industrialization of food, but also suggests how it is becoming easier to find 'real' food again. In the 1970s and 1980s, especially in the United States, you couldn't even find natural yoghurt in the supermarkets. I remember even just a few years ago, living in America and having to find specialist delis to buy real butter – everything in the supermarket was whipped and sweet, urgh.

We have so much good food at our fingertips now, literally if you count ordering your shop online. If you add to that finding local farm shops, markets and delis, then we have a great mix of ingredients and also healthy convenience foods to try.

The weekend before you start your plan, clear out your cupboards, bring all those lovely herbs and spices to the front and think about your cooking. Explore the recipes in this book and your own cookbooks, keeping aware of the Flat Tummy Club plate (see below), and do a big healthy shop for the week ahead. Below, I have included a big list of all the healthy foods and ingredients readily available in most supermarkets. Use this as an initial reminder to write your own. And don't go shopping on an empty stomach because all your healthy intentions will crumble as you wander past the biscuit aisle.

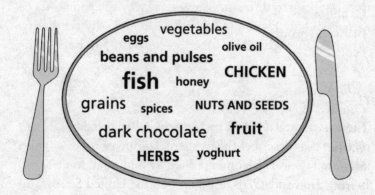

Supermarket Sweep

Fruit and veg

All fruit and vegetables are good, especially whatever is clearly in season and looks/feels freshest.

Greens
Cabbage
Kale
Chard
Cavolo nero
Pak choy
Watercress
Spinach
Lettuces
Broccoli
Cauliflower
Brussels sprouts
Fennel

Allium family
Onion
Leek
Garlic
Shallots
Spring onions
Chives

Root veg
Beetroot
Carrots
Parsnips
Celeriac

Turnip
Swede
Jerusalem artichoke

Above ground
Squashes
Pumpkin
Courgette
Aubergine
Cucumber
Tomato
Peppers
Chillies
Peas
Beans

Fruit
Berries (raspberries, strawberries, blackberries, blueberries, gooseberries, loganberries)
Apples
Pears
Oranges, satsumas, tangerines and clementines
Lemons and limes
Figs
Plums
Peaches
Nectarines
Bananas
Mango
Pineapple
Melon

Fresh herbs and spices
Basil
Mint
Thyme
Parsley
Chives
Rosemary
Sage
Sorrel
Fresh ginger

Extras in the fruit and veg aisle
Stir-fry veg combos for evenings when you have little time
Salads – I've gone off packets of salads, but they are incredibly convenient
Dates
Raw unsalted nuts and seeds

Dairy
Cottage cheese (I recently tried some and I liked it)
Mozzarella
Parmesan (it has such a depth of flavour you only need a little)
Goat's cheese
Natural yoghurt
Butter

Extras in the chilled cabinet
Chilled soups (these seem to be getting better and better, so if you just can't be bothered to make your own every time, don't feel guilty about putting these in your basket)
Smoothies

Deli
Ham
Hummus
Fish pâté (trout, salmon, mackerel)

Meat and fish
Lean cuts of meat
More chicken and turkey than red meat
Go for the freshest looking fish on the counter

Frozen cabinet
Frozen fruit and vegetables still contain all the goodness
and are perfect stand-bys
Fish
Prawns

Staples
Honey – the darker the better
Agave nectar
Dried fruit
Lemon juice
Organic eggs (an omelette can always save a long day at the
office)
Dried or tinned beans and pulses (see page 123 for Cooking
with Beans and Pulses)
Grains (see page 122 for Cooking with Grains)
Olive oil
Balsamic and cider vinegars
Mustards
Olives
Tinned tuna, sardines and mackerel
Noodles and rice

Sesame oil
Soya sauce
Miso soup
Green curry paste
Light coconut milk
Tamarind paste
Capers
Anchovies
Fresh and/or dried stocks
Dried porcini mushrooms
Sea salt
Oats and granola
Oat biscuits
Herbal teas
Dark chocolate

Favourite dried herbs and spices
Ground turmeric
Ground cumin
Paprika
Star anise
Ground coriander
Cloves
Garam masala
Nutmeg
Oregano
Bay leaves
Ground ginger
Mustard seeds
Five-spice powder
Chilli powder

Snacks

A golden Flat Tummy Club rule is to never let yourself get too hungry, as your body will then crave a quick fix in the form of sweets, pastries or biscuits. Make sure you always have plenty of healthy snacks on hand and grab one in the morning and one in the afternoon (just before a commute home is always a good time).

Sweet

- Fresh berries or cherries
- A banana
- A lovely ripe peach or pear
- A fresh fig
- A clementine
- 1 strip of dark chocolate
- Freshly squeezed juice or Innocent smoothie
- Eat Natural bar (not exactly low-calorie, but a great snack for a walk)
- Frozen grapes
- A Prune and Walnut Cookie (see page 373)
- A slice of Dawn's Banana Loaf (see page 369)
- A Dark Chocolate Brownie (see page 374)
- A couple of Nairn's ginger or fruity oat biscuits

Savoury

- Miso soup
- A pot of natural yoghurt
- A good couple of handfuls of seeds
- A good handful of nuts
- ½ an avocado

- Crunchy veg and hummus (my favourite is a simple carrot)
- A couple of slices of ham and a few cherry tomatoes
- A seeded oatcake

Healthy Cooking Tips

- If you love to cook with butter, then I don't recommend cooking with low-fat spreads (urgh), but always look for where you can add healthy flavour instead, for example with herbs, spices, mustards, lemon or lime juice.
- Meat and two veg (one of which is usually potatoes) is traditional, but isn't balanced. The more colourful veg you can get on your plate, the better.
- Don't pile up your plate with pasta, rice or noodles.
- Steaming is ultra healthy and grilling or baking still beats frying.
- Half-fat crème fraîche and 2% Greek yoghurt add creaminess to recipes, but they do curdle more easily, so bring to room temperature and add at the last minute away from the heat.
- Be adventurous and keep trying new recipes. When looking through your cookbooks, think how you can adapt recipes to be healthy *and* tasty. Can you make a creamy dish tomato-based instead?
- The more you cook with less salt, the more your taste buds adapt. Salt cancels out drinking all that water and herbal tea, and too much is no good for anybody. Again, look to herbs and spices for flavour instead.
- Keep an eye on those portions!

Essential kitchen equipment

Blender You don't have to have an expensive food processor, but a blender is essential for making soups.

Steamer Steaming fish and vegetables keeps the nutrients and flavour locked in. I just use an insert that fits on top of a saucepan, but there are also tiered deluxe steamers you can buy if you become a true convert.

Wok Stir-fries are the ultimate quick and easy way to rustle up a delicious supper of fish or chicken and lots of crunchy vegetables with healthy Asian flavours. And when you have growing teenagers to feed, you can simply give them more noodles or rice.

Digital scales Whenever I am unsure of a portion size, I quickly check with the digital scales, for example, what does a 30g portion of cheese actually look like? They help to retrain your brain when it comes to the art of perfect portions.

Microplane grater Excellent for grating lemon zest and ginger but, more importantly, grate cheese really fine so that you feel like you're having a nice mound while only having a tiny bit! Perfect for Parmesan and strong Cheddars (the stronger the taste, the less you need).

Discovering Grains, Beans and Pulses

A few years ago I was inspired to go out and buy the very strange sounding grain (well, technically a grass) quinoa. And that's all I did; it sat at the back of my kitchen cupboard until I realized it was about 18 months out-of-date. When I began my Flat Tummy quest, I decided to be more adventurous with foods I was less familiar with and so I bought more quinoa, discovered it's super simple to cook and soon added it to my repertoire. Similarly, I've never been one for beans and pulses, but now I love to discover new recipes for the array of split peas, lentils and beans of all shapes and sizes you can easily find in the supermarket. If, like me, these ingredients are less familiar to you, I've included a quick rundown of varieties to try and ideas for what to do with them.

Grains

Bulgur wheat is a favourite of mine because it is so easy to cook. You simply pop it in a saucepan, pour over boiling water, add a sprinkle of bouillon and let it sit for 30 minutes. Drain and then heat it when you want to serve up. I like it with saucy dishes like Tarragon Chicken (see page 330) or Smoked Paprika and Sausage Casserole (see page 333).

Couscous is another brilliantly easy stand-by. You just pop it in a bowl, add boiling water so that it just covers the grains and a drizzle of olive oil. Cover with a plate and, after 5 minutes, fluff it up with a fork. Done.

Oats make the perfect breakfast and if you soak them in water overnight or while you have your shower, they soften and you only need a splash of milk for them to taste really creamy.

Pearl barley is fantastic value and perfect for adding to soups and stews; just add the barley to the pot for about 45 minutes of cooking time. Natural home-made Lemon and Ginger Barley Water (see page 223) is also lovely and refreshing.

There are many different types of **rice** available now and I say give them all a try. Many nutritionists favour brown over your standard white rice and there's clearly more roughage in brown than white. But if your digestion is ever in need of a bit of help – whether you are feeling anxious in mind or sensitive in your tummy – then I can personally vouch for the powers of Congee (page 231), a Chinese rice dish that seems to put everything back into balance again.

Beans and pulses

I admit it, I have always associated beans and pulses with bland weirdo health food until I ate a dish at a restaurant called Petersham Nurseries and my eyes were opened to the wonders of the cannellini bean! Since then I have realized that many Mediterranean countries know a thing or two about cooking with beans, as do the South Americans of course. And my favourite dish in Indian restaurants is now dahl. I think it is a good idea to travel around the world within your own kitchen when it comes to beans and pulses. Officially, if you start with dried beans and soak them they will be more nutritious, but the quality of tinned beans has really improved and they are incredibly convenient.

Some beans are also sprouted, particularly alfalfa and mung beans. You can even sprout your own beans, but perhaps that's going a bit far!

Yellow split peas and **red lentils** are perfect for making simple dahls and also adding to stews for an extra dimension (well, to make them go further).

Puy lentils (dark green) are a perfect partner for fish or chicken. They are quite bland on their own, but once you add slow-cooked, caramelized onions, lemon juice and plenty of freshly ground black pepper, they soon perk up.

Adzuki beans, popular in Japan, are a reddish colour and nutty in flavour once cooked. In Chinese medicine, adzuki beans are brilliant for clearing dampness in the body and here in the UK, many of us are prone to damp because of our climate. Damp equals water retention and a feeling of heaviness, so any foods that can help in that department are worth a try.

Mung beans have the most unfortunate name and I can't say I'm in love with them. They tend to be sprouted.

Black beans are popular in South American dishes and work well with robust flavours.

Borlotti beans are lovely and meaty, but not quite as 'in your face' as kidney beans.

There are three types of **haricot beans**. **Cannellini beans** are light in texture, mild-flavoured and often used in Italian dishes. **Flageolet beans**, slightly unripe and green, are a favourite of mine as I don't find them at all overpowering, but nor are they bland. Both are perfect for making Home-made 'Baked' Beans (see page 349). The third is the **common**, or **navy, bean**, which is more often used as the primary ingredient for baked beans.

Butter beans are big, soft and floury and good for absorbing the flavours of spices and herbs.

Kidney beans are strong and meaty and are, of course, the bean of choice in a big pot of chilli.

For me, **chickpeas** either need a delicious curry sauce or should be blitzed into making a delicious Hummus (see page 302). But a tin of chickpeas is also a very handy stand-by for a quick tuna salad.

SWAP TILL YOU DROP

Sandwiches for soups
Cream for 2% Greek yoghurt
Coffee for herbal tea
Potatoes for an alternative vegetable
Mashed potatoes for mashed butternut squash
Biscuits for bananas
Milk chocolate bars for extra dark chocolate
Crisps for oatcakes
Pasta for quinoa, brown rice or bulgur wheat
Salt for herbs (healthy seasoning)
Sweets for berries
Ice cream for freshly squeezed fruit lollies
Creamy curries for tikkas and dahl

Putting It All Together: The Flat Tummy Club 21 Day Plan

THINK ABOUT WHY YOU'D LIKE TO BE SLIMMER, HOW YOU'D LIKE TO LOOK AND FEEL Think about how the pounds might've crept on and learn to be aware of your trigger situations and foods. See yourself, think of the rewards of how you will look and feel.

CHOOSE A QUIET WEEK TO START YOUR PLAN Give your willpower a boost before you get started.

CARRY ON WITH YOUR FOOD, DRINK AND EXERCISE DIARY FOR THE NEXT 21 DAYS Note how you feel as you change your habits. Include your weekly weight with successes from the previous week and challenges you need to think about (lunches, going out with friends, getting home late from the office, travel etc.)

PRINT OFF YOUR GOALS AND YOUR PLAN AND STICK THEM ON THE FRIDGE Focus on all the healthy things you already love and want to try.

PLAN AND PREPARE YOUR WEEK AHEAD WITH MILITARY PRECISION Spend the weekend choosing a few new, and some of your own favourite, healthy recipes for the next few days. Go shopping and stock up on healthy ingredients (see page 114) and plenty of snacks (see page 119). Make a big batch of soup on Sunday and if you know you might get home late during the week, a stew like Vegetarian Chilli (see page 338). The next few pages contain a diary section. Plan as far in advance as you want and then fill out the reality at the end of each day. Really go for it this first week while you create your new healthy habits and give yourself a great start.

KEEP THINGS SIMPLE Start the day with a healthy breakfast, snacks, a big soup for lunch, lots of herbal teas and water, a light supper made with natural, whole foods and some exercise every day, including a lunchtime walk and 10 minutes of Flat Tummy Workout (see page 377).

PUT YOUR EXERCISE IN YOUR WEEKLY PLANNER RIGHT NOW Buy a pedometer to get you started and aim for 10,000 steps a day. If that's easy, increase daily.

THINK BEFORE YOU EAT Whether it's choosing the freshest and most delicious dish on the restaurant menu or saying no thanks when a colleague offers you a big piece of cake.

DON'T GO HUNGRY You don't want your blood sugar to drop and with it your willpower. Get your friends and family on board to cheer you on and not to wave chocolate digestives under your nose.

JOIN THE CLUB to share ideas and keep up your momentum. If you feel a wobble coming on, make a cup of green tea or go and have a bath!

4
GO!

Week One: Banish the Bloat

This is it! I have included three weeks of intense planning to help get you off to a strong start because, as I know from experience, if you can see and feel a difference within the first seven days, and then week by week, you'll be motivated to keep it up.

In the previous preparation chapters, you have: written your food, exercise and drink diary; set your goals; determined the changes you are willing and able to make in your diet and lifestyle to put the Flat Tummy equation back in your favour; plus you've planned and shopped for this first week. Even more importantly, I hope you've spent time boosting your confidence and motivation – seeing in your mind how you're going to look and feel and being honest with yourself about the effort needed to get there.

Banish the Bloat

This week the emphasis is on banishing the bloat – you know, that sluggish, heavy feeling that seems to drag you down in more ways than one. By focusing on strengthening your digestion and flushing out excess water this week, you will shed pounds and also give yourself a big energy boost, just what you need to carry you through these first 21 days and beyond. Whether you are looking to lose quite a bit of weight over time as I did, or you need a quick health kick to feel fit and trim as I do occasionally now I am at my happy weight, the following apply to us all:

- Keep breakfast simple and healthy. During the week have porridge with honey, compote or yoghurt or yoghurt with fresh fruit and a sprinkle of granola. At the weekend, rustle up scrambled or poached eggs with mushrooms or tomatoes (see page 261 for healthy breakfasts and brunches).
- Drink at least six to eight glasses of water/cups of herbal tea through the day. Green tea is excellent for general wellbeing and for a Flat Tummy, so include three or four cups a day.
- If you can, begin the day with a cup of herbal tea or a squeeze of lemon juice in hot water. Dandelion and nettle teas are mild diuretics, which means they help to get rid of excess water. Lemon juice is very support-ive for the digestion and so is also a perfect Flat Tummy start to the day. If you can't function without a cup of tea or coffee first thing, then limit yourself to one cup of coffee or two cups of regular tea in the day and have herbal the rest of the time.
- Choose from the list of healthy snacks for mid-morning and tea time (see page 119).
- Steer clear of bread and enjoy a big soup or salad for lunch. There are lots of ideas in the recipe section (see page 259) or find your local cafés that make their own

soup and offer delicious salads. Ask for the dressing to be on the side wherever possible so that you can just have a little.

- Use the Flat Tummy Club plate (see page 58) as you plan what to have for supper. Replace potatoes with another type of vegetable, include lean proteins (fish and chicken), small portions of whole grains (see page 122) and lots of fresh veg. Include beans (see page 123) in at least three of your meals this week, whether in your lunchtime soup or evening supper. Beans and pulses, and in particular adzuki beans, are excellent for getting rid of excess water, provide lots of fibre and protein and are a real tonic for your digestion.

- Enjoy at least five portions of fruit and vegetables each day.

- Sugar goes straight to your tummy, so steer clear and you'll soon see results. If you have a sweet tooth, replace processed sugary foods with fruit for your snacks or, as I did, have just a couple of pieces of super dark chocolate in the evening or with your afternoon cup of green tea.

- Avoid adding salt to your food as it will tend to absorb excess water just when you want to flush it out.

- Without wanting to get too personal, if you're going to get yourself a flatter tummy, you need to be nicely regular. Include lots of fibre-rich foods in your week: fruit, vegetables, beans and whole grains. If you are not going to the loo at least once a day, then adding a few prunes to your morning porridge can work wonders.

- Do 10 minutes of Flat Tummy Workout (see page 377) each day.

- Fit in at least 30 minutes of exercise a day this week, from a brisk walk at lunchtime to a swim or Pilates class. This is essential for getting your energy flowing as well as combining with your diet changes to put you on the path to a flatter tummy.
- At the beginning and end of each day, and after lunch, take just five minutes to sit quietly and breathe deeply. Let your thoughts come in to your mind, recognize them and then let them gently drift away. As you are making lifestyle changes, think about what went well today and what provided more of a challenge. What can you learn from your reaction?
- Keep up your diary this week. Write in your plan for the day and then the reality – this certainly helps when it comes to willpower and saying 'no thanks'! Remember, the key is for you to make your own positive healthy changes from last week. For some that might mean adding 30 minutes walking a day, while for others who already do lots of exercise, it will be swapping sandwiches and crisps for soup at lunchtime.

I have included my own Flat Tummy Club diary to show you how I put the points above into practice.

The good news is that when you commit to, and carry out, a super healthy first seven days, the results you will see at the end of the week will be just the tonic you need to carry you into the next. I had quite a bit of Christmas indulgence hanging around my middle when I began my own plan, but I was astonished to discover I lost 7lb in seven days, and all the time eating plenty of real food.

More 'banish the bloat' tips

- Eating a small pot of plain natural yoghurt with fruit or a little honey will boost the friendly bacteria in your gut. They improve the digestion, helping you in turn to feel more energetic and get rid of that bloated look and feel.
- Aloe vera juice is very soothing and helps improve the efficiency of your digestive system.
- There are lots of herbs and spices that are good for digestion. Cardamom can help with flatulence while cinnamon aids a dodgy tummy (technical term) and may help a little with IBS. Others include cumin, fennel and ginger. Lemon balm is good both for digestion and stress – what a great combination. And you probably know peppermint as a digestive tonic, but interestingly it's even better to drink before you eat, rather than after.
- A full body aromatherapy massage or reflexology can do wonders for getting your digestion going.
- If you feel like you might have a bit of trapped wind, then a walk is a great way to get it moving and released.
- Don't rush your food. Eating slowly and in a relaxed frame of mind means that you will digest the food more effectively and prevent bloating or wind.

KATE'S DAY 1

On rising: Cup of nettle tea

Breakfast: Porridge with agave syrup (½ water, ½ semi-skimmed milk)

Snack: Miso soup

Lunch: Smoked salmon, avocado, grilled chicken, salad (no dressing because Day 1 and feeling strong!)

Snack: Clementine

Dinner: Butternut Squash and Pear Soup (see page 274), strip of of dark chocolate

Drinks: 3 x cups of green tea, 5 x glasses of water

Exercise: 15,000 steps (about 1 ½ hours walking to and from the train station), 10 minutes of Flat Tummy Workout (see page 377)

Tip of the day A couple of squares of dark chocolate is not only good for you, but also feels like a little treat or ritual at the end of the day, savoured with a cup of herbal tea. It's important to feel you are treating yourself as you're putting so much effort in, whether it's lots of luxurious baths, disappearing into your bedroom to read a book or listen to your favourite music or some delicious dark chocolate.

YOUR DAY 1

On rising:
....

Breakfast:
....

....

Snack:
....

Lunch:
....

....

Snack:
....

Dinner:
....

....

Drinks:
....

Exercise:
....

KATE'S DAY 2

On rising: Cup of nettle tea

Breakfast: Porridge with agave syrup

Snack: Clementine

Lunch: Big vegetable and chickpea soup from Leon, flatbread

Snack: Small pot of natural yoghurt

Dinner: Herb, mushroom and Parmesan Omelette (see page 309), strip of dark chocolate

Drinks: 3 x cups of green tea, 4 x glasses of water

Exercise: 15,000 steps, 10 minutes of Flat Tummy Workout (see page 377)

Tip of the day Clementines were one of my 'saviours', something I could easily grab and keep on hand for whenever I got peckish. For you it might be apples, bananas, nuts or a pot of yoghurt – the key is for these foods to be things you really like rather than trying to eat them purely because they are 'good for you'.

YOUR DAY 2

On rising:
....

Breakfast:
....

....

Snack:
....

Lunch:
....

....

Snack:
....

Dinner:
....

....

Drinks:
....

Exercise:
....

KATE'S DAY 3

On rising: Cup of dandelion tea

Breakfast: Porridge with Quick-and-Easy Berry Compote (see page 264)

Snack: Banana

Lunch: Big broccoli and Stilton soup

Snack: Eat Natural with . . . Almonds, Apricots and a Yoghurt Coating bar

Dinner: Spicy Chicken, Fennel and Tomato (see page 326)

Drinks: 3 x cups of green tea, 1 x cup of nettle tea, 3 x glasses of water

Exercise: 14,000 steps (one way to the train station and a walk at lunchtime), 10 minutes of Flat Tummy Workout (see page 377)

Tip of the day Spices improve your digestion, which in turn helps lead to a flatter tummy. Plus the more flavour you can add to your dishes, the more you can savour each mouthful rather than eating too much, too quickly. Remember, don't hoover up your dinner and stop when you are two thirds full – there is a time delay between your stomach signalling it is full and your brain receiving the message.

YOUR DAY 3

On rising:

....

Breakfast:

....

....

Snack:

....

Lunch:

....

....

Snack:

....

Dinner:

....

....

Drinks:

....

Exercise:

....

KATE'S DAY 4

On rising: Lemon juice and hot water
Breakfast: Porridge with Quick-and-Easy Berry Compote
   (see page 264)
Snack: Banana
Lunch: Ham and cabbage soup, flatbread
Snack: Miso soup
Dinner: Monkfish Stew with Warming Herbs and Spices
   (see page 320), strip of dark chocolate
Drinks: 3 x cups of herbal tea, 3 x glasses of water

Exercise: 15,000 steps, 10 minutes of Flat Tummy
   Workout (see page 377)

Tip of the day The more green leafies you can cram into
your day the more densely packed in nutrients your diet will
be. Our bodies absorb the highest concentration of vitamins
and minerals from green vegetables with hardly any calories
and lots of fibre for our digestion. They are the ultimate flat
tummy food.

YOUR DAY 4

On rising:
....

Breakfast:
....

....

Snack:
....

Lunch:
....

....

Snack:
....

Dinner:
....

....

Drinks:
....

Exercise:
....

KATE'S DAY 5

On rising: Cup of green tea

Breakfast: Porridge with soft prunes and a little honey

Snack: Innocent smoothie

Lunch: Leon superfood salad (see page 292 for a home-made version)

Snack: Another smoothie (got caught out hungry on the way home – forgot to take fruit to work)

Dinner: Tarragon Chicken (see page 330) with purple sprouting broccoli, couple of squares of dark chocolate

Drinks: Lots of herbal tea and water during the day

Exercise: 16,500 steps, 10 minutes of Flat Tummy Workout (see page 377)

Tip of the day If you struggle to get on with fruit, then try an Innocent smoothie, which counts as two of your five a day. These drinks contain nothing but fruit, squished up for your convenience.

YOUR DAY 5

On rising:
....

Breakfast:
....

....

Snack:
....

Lunch:
....

....

Snack:
....

Dinner:
....

....

Drinks:
....

Exercise:
....

KATE'S DAY 6

On rising: Lemon juice and hot water

Breakfast: Granola, natural yoghurt, berries and banana

Snack: Handful of dried apricots

Lunch: Celeriac, Wild Mushroom and Rosemary Soup (see page 271), 3 oatcakes and some Brie (I specifically went to the deli so I could buy just enough for lunch rather than a big wedge that I'd be tempted to polish off)

Snack: Eat Natural bar

Dinner: Tarragon Chicken (made double yesterday) with bulgur wheat and purple sprouting broccoli

Drinks: 6 x cups of herbal tea

Exercise: 10,000 steps, 10 minutes of Flat Tummy Workout (see page 377)

Tip of the day Oatcakes are a good friend of the Flat Tummy Club. When you are trying to eat less bread, they provide the perfect natural alternative and now come in many varieties for when you need a quick and healthy snack. Nairn's are a favourite because they even do snack packs and their ginger oatcakes are just what you need to curb the urge for a chocolate digestive.

YOUR DAY 6

On rising:
....

Breakfast:
....

....

Snack:
....

Lunch:
....

....

Snack:
....

Dinner:
....

....

Drinks:
....

Exercise:
....

KATE'S DAY 7

On rising: Lemon juice and hot water

Breakfast: Porridge with soft prunes and a little honey (again)

Snack: Banana, pain au chocolat (I decided I would have a treat)

Lunch: Celeriac, Wild Mushroom and Rosemary Soup from yesterday, walnut roll

Snack: Eat Natural bar

Dinner: Tuna Stir-Fry (see page 318), clementine

Treat: Drinks: 6 x cups of herbal tea

Exercise: 18,000 steps, 10 minutes of Flat Tummy Workout (see page 377)

Tip of the day Wanting to treat yourself at the end of a really good week is completely normal, after all we're only human, but as I was still in the early days of losing weight I didn't really enjoy my Sunday pain au chocolat. Now I realize it would've been better to wait a bit until I was feeling more in balance with myself. However, I didn't dwell on it; I went for a nice Sunday afternoon walk and prepared for Week Two.

YOUR DAY 7

On rising:
....

Breakfast:
....

....

Snack:
....

Lunch:
....

....

Snack:
....

Dinner:
....

....

Drinks:
....

Exercise:
....

Week Two: Momentum and Motivation

So how did the first week go? What went well for you, which meals were your favourites and did you discover you quite enjoy exercise after all? I was on a bit of a high after my first week because it was literally the first full healthy week I had had in over three years. I anticipated feeling dreadful as a result, but I had more energy, I stopped hitting the snooze button in the morning and I simply felt good.

Use this momentum to literally propel you into the next week. If you feel ever so slightly smug because you're not drinking alcohol, go with it. If you can't seem to stop telling people what you're doing, great, this is a really good sign things are going well. Momentum equals motivation and you can both look back over the past week and look forward to keeping going.

If this week of healthy eating and living has been a bit of a shock to your system, you might be having headaches, sense you have a cold coming on and generally feel a bit rubbish. This is quite a challenge to get through, but the good news is that these are all signs of your body healing and cleansing itself. Make sure you drink plenty of water and herbal tea to keep well hydrated and if at all possible, keep your weekend as free as possible to relax, go for lovely walks and prepare for the week ahead.

After the initial burst of the first week, carrying on through the weekend and into the next week can test our motivation. Our healthy habits are far from ingrained at this time, so I say don't put them through tests that are too tough. If you often meet friends in the pub on a Friday night or for Sunday lunch and you're worried you won't be able to resist a few drinks, then why not suggest going out for dinner instead? I remember in my second week going out for an Indian. I was worried all my good work would be undone with one pasanda, rice, naan and beer, but because I steeled my nerve before I arrived, I looked carefully and with much more interest than usual at the menu and discovered a lemony chicken tikka (the one that comes out sizzling from the grill rather than in a sauce) and chose two vegetables to go with it. I promise, it was more delicious than anything I'd had in that restaurant before, and it's one of my favourite local haunts (see page 222 for lots of tips on eating out).

Getting Through the Weekend

Don't take your eye off the ball over the weekend, but spend some time planning, preparing and cooking for the week ahead, along with a couple of big walks. While you are reconnecting with the inner healthy you, keep these points in mind:

- Get away from seeing the weekend as an excuse or opportunity to binge in the name of rewarding yourself for a tough week. I don't mean have no fun, I promise, but while you are creating healthy habits, keep a balance between the work week and the weekend.

- Do book in treats like going to the cinema, out for dinner or book a spa day with friends.
- Plan and shop for the week ahead, making sure you are stocked up on all the healthy foods you are enjoying.
- Cook up a batch of soup or a big pot of stew that makes Monday dinner a cinch.
- For a healthy roast dinner, go for roast chicken with roasted carrots (instead of potatoes) and green veggies.

Motivation Exercises

CHART YOUR PROGRESS It is a good idea to weigh yourself every Sunday morning at the same time as this is the perfect day to spend a little time charting and reflecting on your progress. I would often go for a long walk on Sundays and so I'd get my fix of vitamin D from hours of being outside, burn off lots of calories, get fit and plan some healthy meals for the next week all at the same time. Chart your progress in your food diary. Don't limit this to how many pounds you have lost, but also whether you are feeling less bloated or more energetic.

I remember I was asked by a magazine to write the two things that I do every day to try and keep healthy. This is a great exercise to do now. What are just two things from last week that you really enjoyed and want to fit into your every day?

THE TWO THINGS I LOVE DOING EVERY DAY . . .
Walking: It's a small thing, but is making all the difference
for me. Whether it's along the river or just between tube
stations, it clears my head, relaxes me and I just love being
outside, so it's an all round tonic that is also helping to
make me slim and healthy. I remembered how much I loved
to walk when some friends and I signed up for a charity
trek in Nepal, the trek was the perfect goal to create a
healthy habit that I now love to fit into my day.
Cooking: I had become such a lazy cook, but now that I'm
planning my meals and shopping, I'm enjoying both the
cooking and eating the fruits of my labour.

RECOGNIZE YOUR LIMITATIONS This might strike
you as a little negative, but it's important because unchecked
positive thinking often raises our expectations to unrealistic heights, and then we feel like a failure when they don't
magically materialize. It's a fine balance between not being
too tough on yourself, but also making real changes that
will lead to the difference you desire.

DON'T LET A LAPSE GO ON TO THE NEXT DAY
Tomorrow is another day, but don't make the mistake of
saying that again tomorrow!

PICTURE YOUR GOAL Find a lovely picture of yourself
that sums up the way you'd like to look and feel and pop it
somewhere you can see it every day. Or simply find a
gorgeous photograph of where you're going on holiday if
that's your goal. I make myself a diary through one of those
online personal printing companies each year that has a
photograph of fresh, healthy ingredients on each page,
from a mass of purple sprouting broccoli to a crate of

strawberries. It definitely helps to keep me in the Flat Tummy mood.

FIRE UP YOUR INSPIRATION 'Diets' are often extremely boring. We hold out for as long as our initial willpower lasts and then we fall off the wagon in spectacular fashion, just so relieved to be free again. This is why I say make your *own* changes and your own plan because Flat Tummy Club is about feeling fired up and inspired, both from within and also from all around you. If you have a smartphone, explore all the free recipe apps (my favourite is Epicurious) or Google what to do with an ingredient. Buy a book of local walks. And keep your eyes open as you shop for foods that look particularly good – a lovely pineapple might take your fancy or you might spot the first asparagus of the season.

REWARDS ...

Are your rewards, treats and comforts often food related? Have a think about all the other things that also make you feel good, from meeting a friend for coffee to going for a run (honest, for a friend of mine running is what makes her feel great) to a relaxing evening bath with lots of luxurious bath oils. Also, think about the rewards of how you will feel when you reach your goal – looking slim in that new dress with radiant skin and bright eyes or feeling confident and energized.

At the end of my second week, I combined a food treat with a really healthy activity. I went for a long walk in the Surrey Hills (and included a couple of steep climbs for good measure) and enjoyed a bacon sandwich at the start. Somehow I think it tastes even better when you are out in the open air and about to spend four hours in the spectacular countryside.

... AND RITUALS

We often think only of our negative or unhealthy habits, but we all have positive and healthy rituals too and it's worth jotting these down for the next few weeks. If your healthy habits have gone out of the window recently, then this is the perfect time to put them back into your day. Do you love a quiet and peaceful cup of herbal tea in the afternoon, for example, or a walk outside at lunchtime? Rituals are very calming, and as stress is no friend to the Flat Tummy (see page 179) they are perfect for gently strengthening your resolve and distracting you from temptations.

Tales from the Club

A friend posted on Facebook yesterday that she hadn't had time to go food shopping before lunch and had to resort to the dreaded cuppa soup. As someone who works at home, I know this depressing realization all too well. The morning flies by, suddenly you are starving and you're scrabbling around for an old tin of tuna or a ryvita. I did slightly, but only slightly, better yesterday when I discovered all I had that was easy for lunch was an avocado, a couple of oatcakes and my version of cuppa soup, miso soup. It wasn't so boring after all, with some basil and balsamic on the avocado and a Yeo Valley yoghurt for afters.

Fortunately the weather brightened up right at the end of the day, so I managed to get outside for some exercise right when I would usually pour myself a glass of wine.

I will not lie – getting in healthy habits again is an effort. But I am feeling very clear-headed and I'm getting more work done and seem to be feeling quite positive . . .

Finding Flat Tummy Time

'Finding time' is one of the hardest challenges when trying to be healthy or lose weight and it's the most common challenge that comes up in my Flat Tummy conversations. Somehow, stressful long days at work or demands from family life knock us off our stride in the blink of an eye. As a nation, we work the longest hours in Europe and for many people you can add an hour's commute at either end of the day, so we're rushed in the morning and shattered in the evening. One woman described her average day to me and there wasn't even a break for lunch, just a few sandwiches and crisps as part of the meeting, and of course those endless cups of coffee to try and keep alert when what you really need is a breath of fresh air and to get your body moving.

It's easy to see the links between feeling like you don't have any time to grabbing whatever food is available, whether it's healthy or not, to then feeling a bit lacklustre and like you don't have the energy to get everything done in the day, so the pressures on your time become even greater. I must admit, I work freelance now and so I do have more time in general, but I began my 'transformation' while I was still at work in a full-time job, so I had to start prioritizing my health in order to find the time I needed for healthy shopping, cooking and the big one, exercising.

I think we all have individual time challenges and we all have to be pretty savvy to get those 24 hours in the day to work for, rather than against, us. A friend of mine has two children under three and I realized when I went to stay with her while her husband was away that she uses every single minute of the day. Her healthy goals are simple, but by no means easy. Firstly, she has banished ready meals and convenience foods and so cooks every meal from scratch. And secondly, she gets out for a walk and some fresh air with the two little ones every day. When I visited, after the mini marathon of putting the children to bed, my friend roasted a pheasant and made the most delicious creamed leeks. The next day, in the gap between dropping her two-year-old off at nursery and feeding the baby, she made Chilled Apple Soup (see page 285 for the recipe). As you can tell, I wasn't exactly pulling my weight, so I pitched in with Vegetarian Chilli that evening (see page 338) and, following my friend's instructions, made enough to last her another couple of meals at least.

My friend has a weekly planner on the kitchen pin board and plans meals for the family so that she can order a big shop online. She also deliberately makes double the portions quite often so that she has two meals for the effort of one. You'd think perhaps she might get into a rut of doing the same meals all the time this way, but my friend loves to rummage through her recipe files when she has a spare few minutes with a cup of tea and try new recipes or rediscover old favourites long forgotten.

Here are some ideas for how to have more time, or at least the perception of it. The benefits are not only for the body, but also for the mind and, dare I say it, the soul.

- Have a look at your day – what's stealing your time, where are the slivers or chunks that you can reclaim?
- You are likely do this anyway, but use your commute time to either relax (but then be active when you get home) or plan and make lists that will benefit your Flat Tummy (don't get caught with an empty fridge and end up eating a loaf of bread and butter) and your time (be ultra efficient at work the next day as you tick off your list).
- Think about how much time you spend watching the television and on the web. Before you cry that life without *The Apprentice* wouldn't be worth living, think about the rubbish you also watch and could definitely live without.
- I don't want to get too deep, but think about how you are prioritizing your life and how far down the list your health is right now. If it's at the top (why else would you join the Club?), then brilliant, use that motivation to find more time, right now.
- Do you find it hard to say no? No? Then you're lucky, because this is an excellent way to find time and the confidence to be master of your own destiny. If the thought of saying no sends you into a panic that your manager won't think you're working as hard as possible or you'll just end up having an argument with your partner or children, then you're not alone, this is really

hard. There is likely to be someone you know who is a master of this and it's worth doing a bit of watching and learning. Practise with small things and build up as you get the hang of it.

- How many hours can you honestly work productively for during an average day? What are you doing with the downtime? Are you 'sort of working', not really achieving much? Could you go for a 15-minute walk instead? Or if your life is timed to the minute, then make appointments for healthy stuff in your diary and on your lists!

- Learn from friends. I know someone who is just terrible at leaving work on time, but is committed to her daily run and so has stopped wasting so much time in the morning, finding the half hour she needs. Another friend has a baby and just couldn't work out how to find time to work out until she discovered Buddha Baby, yoga for you and your baby.

- Tell people you are on the lookout for more time. Get family, friends and even managers on side. Frame it positively, so it's not about doing less work or spending less time with the kids, but it is about wanting to be more effective all round. People who manage time better are less stressed and more effective, so your bosses and your loved ones win in the end anyway.

- Take small steps, but put yourself at the top of the list for once. And put healthy things you love doing/eating at the top of the list too, rather than things that feel more like a punishment.

KATE'S DAY 8

On rising: Cup of nettle tea

Breakfast: Porridge with Quick-and-Easy Berry Compote (see page 264)

Snack: Pear

Lunch: Beetroot and fennel salad, rabbit, vegetables and small gnocchi (restaurant lunch)

Snack: Nairns ginger oatcake with green tea

Dinner: Beetroot and Apple Soup (see page 273), walnut roll

Drinks: 3 x cups of green tea, 3 x glasses of water, 1 x cup of coffee

Exercise: Tae Bo workout

Tip of the day If you are going out to eat, use it as the perfect opportunity to order lots of lovely side vegetables. A substantial lunch also means you can have a light supper of soup or a salad, which will be nice and easy on your tummy.

YOUR DAY 8

On rising:
....

Breakfast:
....

....

Snack:
....

Lunch:
....

....

Snack:
....

Dinner:
....

....

Drinks:
....

Exercise:
....

KATE'S DAY 9

On rising: Lemon juice and hot water

Breakfast: Porridge with Quick-and-Easy Berry Compote (see page 264)

Snack: Innocent smoothie

Lunch: Octopus carpaccio and salad, red mullet and fennel, cucumber, crème fraîche and greens (restaurant lunch)

Snack: Nairns ginger oatcake

Dinner: Beetroot and Apple Soup (I made double) with three cheesy Nairn's

Drinks: 3 x cups of green tea, 4 x glasses of water, water with lime juice (in the restaurant – delicious), 1 x cup of fresh mint tea

Exercise: 20,000 steps, 10 minutes of Flat Tummy Workout (see page 377)

Tip of the day Fresh mint tea is refreshing and excellent for the digestion; it is also a lovely ritual to make a pot of fresh tea rather than always dunk a tea bag. You can even keep a pot of mint on your desk or your windowsill and simply pick a few leaves when you fancy a cuppa.

YOUR DAY 9

On rising:
....

Breakfast:
....

....

Snack:
....

Lunch:
....

....

Snack:
....

Dinner:
....

....

Drinks:
....

Exercise:
....

KATE'S DAY 10

On rising: Cup of green tea
Breakfast: Granola, natural yoghurt and raspberries
Snack: Miso soup
Lunch: Mushroom risotto soup from Pret A Manger
Snack: Eat Natural bar, clementine
Dinner: Lemon chicken tikka, spinach, mushrooms and
    dahl (shared at the Indian restaurant)
Drinks: 1 glass of red wine, 3 x cups of green tea, 1 x
    cup of nettle tea, 3 x glasses of water

Exercise: 18,000 steps, 10 minutes of Flat Tummy
    Workout (see page 377)

Tip of the day Putting grains in your soups adds nutrition
and makes them even more satisfying. With simple vegetable
soups, enjoy a flatbread or a couple of oatcakes. If you can
regularly enjoy soup as one of your daily meals, you will
definitely notice the difference.

YOUR DAY 10

On rising:

....

Breakfast:

....

....

Snack:

....

Lunch:

....

....

Snack:

....

Dinner:

....

....

Drinks:

....

Exercise:

....

KATE'S DAY 11

On rising: Cup of dandelion tea

Breakfast: Porridge with a sprinkle of cinnamon and a little honey

Snack: Clementine, 2 cheesy oatcakes

Lunch: Beetroot and Feta Couscous (see page 305)

Snack: Strip of dark chocolate

Dinner: Lemon and Herb Chicken (see page 325) with sautéed onions and chard, small pot of natural yoghurt with a drizzle of honey

Drinks: 3 x cups of herbal tea, 3 x glasses of water, 1 x cup of green tea

Exercise: 17,000 steps, 10 minutes of Flat Tummy Workout (see page 377)

Tip of the day Going for a walk every day at lunchtime is both a great exercise habit and helps you to feel relaxed and refreshed for the afternoon, especially if you are working hard. You may feel you don't have the time, but your mind will work so much more effectively as a result and you'll get even more done than if you try to work through. And don't eat while working as your brain is needed for good digestion.

YOUR DAY 11

On rising:
....

Breakfast:
....

....

Snack:
....

Lunch:
....

....

Snack:
....

Dinner:
....

....

Drinks:
....

Exercise:
....

KATE'S DAY 12

On rising: Cup of dandelion tea
Breakfast: Porridge with honey and cinnamon
Snack: ½ Eat Natural bar
Lunch: Beeetroot and Feta couscous (made double
yesterday for lunch)
Snack: Innocent smoothie
Dinner: Sea Bass and Lemony Leeks (see page 314)
Drinks: Lots of herbal tea and water during the day

Exercise: 8,000 steps, 10 minutes of Flat Tummy Workout
(see page 377)

Tip of the day Beware the office feeder. These are the kind-hearted, generous souls who offer biscuits and treats and say 'go on, who cares' and the like. Be upfront and honest and ask them to help you out in your Flat Tummy quest.

YOUR DAY 12

On rising:
....

Breakfast:
....

....

Snack:
....

Lunch:
....

....

Snack:
....

Dinner:
....

....

Drinks:
....

Exercise:
....

KATE'S DAY 13

On rising:

Breakfast: Porridge with Quick-and-Easy Berry Compote (see page 264)

Snack: Breakfast Muffin (see page 263, baked by a friend and delicious)

Lunch: Leek, pancetta and Parmesan Omelette (see page 309)

Snack: Miso soup, an apple

Dinner: Smoked Paprika and Sausage Casserole (see page 333) with cabbage

Drinks: 6 x cups of herbal tea (struggled to drink water away from the office)

Exercise: Over 20,000 steps (3 hours' walk), 10 minutes of Flat Tummy Workout (see page 377)

Tip of the day Use the weekend to relax and also fire up your food senses. Find out if there is a market or farm shop near you, or jot down a few recipe ideas for the week ahead. Make a big batch of soup and a stew that will give you a head start for Monday.

YOUR DAY 13

On rising:
....

Breakfast:
....

....

Snack:
....

Lunch:
....

....

Snack:
....

Dinner:
....

....

Drinks:
....

Exercise:
....

KATE'S DAY 14

On rising: Cup of green tea
Breakfast: Porridge with honey
Snack: Small bacon roll (at start of big walk)
Lunch: Chicken and bulgur wheat, banana, clementine
and a flask of green tea for my picnic
Snack: Innocent smoothie
Dinner: Vegetarian Chilli (see page 331), strip of dark
chocolate
Drinks: Plenty of herbal tea

Exercise: 7½ miles walking and two steep hills!

Tip of the day Go for a good long walk every weekend and
you'll tip the Flat Tummy balance firmly in your favour, while
clearing your head for the start of the week. If you can't then
best to leave out the bacon rolls.

YOUR DAY 14

On rising:
....

Breakfast:
....

....

Snack:
....

Lunch:
....

....

Snack:
....

Dinner:
....

....

Drinks:
....

Exercise:
....

Week Three: The Wall

Welcome to Week Three. The good news is that by now your body is beginning to be on your side, your healthy snacks are keeping your blood sugar nice and balanced and you don't physically crave the sugary fixes (although for women who are premenstrual this week, see page 241). By this time I was feeling great, but I did have to work on my willpower and my mental cravings to keep on my path to a Flat Tummy.

JOT DOWN ALL THE BENEFITS OF THE LAST COUPLE OF WEEKS Physical, emotional and mental. Do you have more energy, are you more focused at work or cooking delicious meals?

THINK AGAIN OF YOUR GOALS How do you feel right now and how will you feel as you reach your goals. Continue to chart your progress and write down a few notes to help set your intentions again for this week. Which changes to your diet or lifestyle are you feeling really good about? The great news is that these can happily stay with you for life.

BOOK IN A WEEKEND DETOX (see page 226) Find a quiet weekend for a healthy boost.

REMEMBER TO KEEP THINGS SIMPLE Stock up on the healthy foods you know you love and give anything processed or full of additives a wide berth.

GOING OUT TO EAT CAN OFTEN SEEM LIKE A CHALLENGE However, welcome these treats as opportunities to find fresh and delicious looking dishes on the menu (see page 222 for more restaurant tips).

HAVE YOU CUT DOWN ON ALCOHOL FOR YOUR PLAN? If so, ask yourself how confident you feel about going to the pub and 'just having one' or savouring a glass of wine with dinner occasionally. Listen to your instincts and also learn from the experience, whether you kept to your new way of thinking or had a lapse.

DID YOU START OUT SLOWLY WITH EXERCISE IN WEEKS ONE AND TWO? Up the ante this week, from 30 minutes walking a day to 45 minutes, for example.

How to Deal with Cravings

We all experience cravings for our nemesis foods on occasion. Sometimes these are physical cravings, especially for women at certain times of the month (see page 241) or when we are stressed (see page 179), and often they are mental cravings. For many people, food has various emotional attachments: sweets equal a reward or comfort, cake equals 'treat'. It's no surprise that we grow up seeing particular foods as a comfort. For my friend, it's a tub of ice cream and for me it is crisps and cheese and Marmite sandwiches because I was a fussy eater as a child, but could always rely on this combination to feel in my comfort zone. By placing the emphasis on finding the healthy foods we love rather than fixating on giving up all of our 'favourite things' we gradually loosen that emotional attachment, or craving. Personally, I have made a very conscious effort to now associate a glass of wine with something delicious to enjoy and savour rather than grasp and crave at the end of a stressful day. I have found that both my body and mind can play a part when it comes to seeing off a craving:

Body

As you change your diet and exercise more, your body craves the quick fixes less and less over time. It likes being in balance and doesn't want the acute highs and lows that it was once addicted to. And the more you can keep your blood sugar balanced by eating regularly through the day, the less you will be physically drawn to high-sugar fixes.

Mind

Whenever you are faced with a craving, just stop for a minute and think it through. Where's it come from and how will you feel afterwards if you eat that entire packet of biscuits? Can you distract and comfort yourself with an alternative treat like a luxurious bath or even just put on your trainers and go round the block?

I can't say I never give in to cravings; I'm a normal human being and modern life doesn't exactly make it easy. But I have become much better at taking a moment and making a healthier choice, and feeling all the better for it.

Excuses, Excuses

There is often a point while making new healthy habits that our old, less healthy ones get into our psyche and start to make a nuisance of themselves. We might be feeling tired or have had a bad day; sometimes we're just not sure if we can be bothered to keep making the effort and the little devil on our shoulder asks is it really worth it. My mum is hilarious when it comes to excuses, and we all have a few of these tucked up our sleeve. Have a think about your own and then look at them from the alternative perspective; see if you can turn a negative into a positive.

20 excuses to give up . . .

1. I'm just getting older and fatter, that's life
2. I'm miserable when I'm on a 'diet'
3. Cake is my only vice
4. I'm single
5. I'm married
6. I have kids
7. I don't want to change my life for the sake of losing weight
8. I can't cook
9. It's no fun
10. I hate healthy food
11. I don't have time to exercise
12. It's Christmas/my birthday
13. It's the holidays
14. I'm stressed
15. Being healthy is boring
16. I love chocolate too much
17. I'm not really bothered
18. I must have the fat gene
19. I don't have any willpower
20. Because I might fail

On the other hand . . .

1. My mum was determined that she was just getting older and fatter until she decided to give it a go. With a few changes she's now feeling younger and slimmer!

2. Yes, the words 'I'm on a diet' are often synonymous with 'I'm fed up'. I swear I didn't say this on purpose, but when a friend noticed I was looking slimmer, I replied, 'I've been taking better care of myself'. Okay, you might think I'm just incredibly smug, but it's true.

3. A friend of mine is such a lovely person and cake really is her only vice, plus she is a brilliant baker. We are now channelling her cooking skills into creating healthier alternatives and making the cakes an extra special treat.

4. Who cares if you look good naked? You do!

5. See Point 4.

6. You will soon inspire your children to be healthy and active by practising what you preach.

7. You don't have to eat mung beans, sachets of diet shakes or never go to the pub again to be more healthy. But change is really good for us, even small changes.

8. I'm not much of a cook, but learning is so enjoyable, and when you produce something delicious, you feel fantastic.

9. We don't exactly grow up thinking that 'being good' is much fun; they don't call them 'guilty' pleasures for nothing.

10. We don't exactly grow up thinking that healthy food is yummy and delicious either.

11. How much time do you spend watching the television?

12. Pick your battles. Christmas or your birthday is no time to eat cabbage soup, but look for treats that pack a

small, but intense punch rather than devouring an entire tin of Celebrations.

13. You have time on holiday to remind your senses to really savour food and mealtimes and choose interesting new foods. Ask what is super fresh, authentic and local and don't fall into old habits like piling on the pastries at the breakfast buffet!

14. We crave comfort in times of stress (see page 179) and so it is a physical as well as mental challenge to stay healthy. If you can manage to stand back from the feelings of stress for a moment and choose simple, healthy foods, then you will cope so much more effectively. Rather than feel a blow to your confidence, you will also help to nurture that inner strength. It is definitely not easy, but maybe ask a friend to help and be the voice of reason as you reach for a second cream cake or bottle of wine!

15. It's easy to rely on just a few core foods so that we can lose weight, and then once boredom sets in, we revert back to our old habits. Always be on the lookout for new ingredients and recipes, do a different workout or walk a new route. And of course, for lots of ideas just sign up to Flat Tummy Club News.

16. Once you develop a taste for dark chocolate, you never look back.

17. I slipped back and forth between wanting to be healthy and couldn't be bothered for about three years, so I definitely know how that feels! If apathy begins to set in, try going back to writing a food and mood diary, get your brain engaged again with how you want to feel healthier, more energetic and really enjoy walking up and down the beach in your bikini. Ask around for inspiration because we've all been there.

18. We absolutely all come in different shapes and sizes and for many of us, even if we feel and look in the best shape of our life, the nurse in our local surgery will frown as we step onto the scales. The key is to be honest with ourselves and be aware of when being a few pounds over our ideal is drifting towards feeling rather uncomfortable.

19. Willpower is a tricky customer. As soon as our brains are busy doing things like work, our willpower diminishes (see page 36). Exercise it like a muscle, so every time you have a choice about what to eat or whether to go to the gym or walk to work, stop for a moment, think through what's really the best option for you and then go for it.

20. Feel the fear and do it anyway.

Tales from the Club
You know, those habits I had before I lost the weight are still ready to pounce at any time . . . in fact, they have. For me, it's wine, cheese and morning croissants. The past couple of weeks have been a bit of a slippery slope and so it's time to take it in hand.

Yesterday I went for a long walk to help balance out the weekend excesses and I created a little corner of healthi-ness in my kitchen to remind me of my good intentions this morning. This includes porridge, a box of green tea, flax-seed oil capsules and a simple note – five-a-day, water and herbal tea, no wine until Friday!

It's not quite Gwyneth's regime for getting into shape for Ironman 2 and I am not going to be making myself a kale juice any time soon. I say keep it simple, and for me that's homing in on less bread, less booze, more fruit and veg. If I had fallen out of the exercise habit, I would focus on that, or if I were sneaking choc bars, I'd think how to replace them. The key is to think of the benefits, not the hardship! Even a glass of wine nowadays makes me a little less energetic in the morning, so I look forward to finding it easier to get up this week. I love fruit and veg, but I am a bit lazy to be honest so I do need to make an effort to get more into my day. And drinking lots of water and herbal tea will likely refresh my system, make me feel better and might even make me look radiant . . . OK, I am stretching it now, but even as I type I'm feeling good rather than fed up at the prospect. What are your keys to a healthy week? I do think writing them down and then working out how to adapt to the various challenges of the week really helps – be realistic and optimistic! First step, cup of green tea . . .

Keeping Healthy When STRESSED!!!!!!!!

If you are anything like me, then you find it's all too easy to let your healthy intentions go haywire when stressed and very busy, even though it tends to just make things worse. I remember working on a book all about healthy eating and found the deadlines so stressful my own diet deteriorated rapidly. I'd be 'too busy and tired' to cook, so resort to ready meals and evening picnics comprised of all my nemesis foods (bread, cheese, wine). And as I was fed up being so busy, I then felt the need for treats (cake, wine).

The reason stress is so often associated with making poor food choices is that it interferes with our adrenals. The adrenals secrete adrenalin to provide us with energy, which when everything is in a happy balance, all works smoothly and we have a healthy appetite. However, when we are stressed our body goes into 'fight or flight' mode and secretes more adrenalin, hence signalling the need for more food as fuel. This was very handy back when we had to run away from wild animals on a daily basis, but the problem with most modern-day stress is that it is emotional rather than physical. We don't actually need the extra calories, but we still crave them. Hence those with a sweet tooth end up eating a tub of Ben & Jerry's while the rest of us eat a family pack of crisps or pizza for four.

Is this you?
Recognizing the signs of stress is the first helpful step to coping with it and curbing your cravings.

- Constantly feeling tired
- You avoid things that clearly need doing, you're not sure why, but it only makes matters worse
- You feel tense in your body, which can lead to headaches, shoulder, neck and back aches, upset stomach
- Either you struggle to get a good night's sleep or you are sleeping too much and can't seem to get up in the morning
- Some people lose their appetite, while others reach out for all their 'comfort foods'
- You feel like you have too much to get through in the day and panic about the lack of time, but ironically lack the motivation to really get going
- You find it difficult to focus, like your mind is all over the place, going at a hundred miles an hour; you can't concentrate
- You might feel under quite a bit of pressure

It's tough because when we are stressed, we don't feel we have any time or energy to do something about it, so the last thing we want to take away is that bit of comfort in a bar of Galaxy or a glass of wine. When I read articles on how to manage stress, it all seems very logical, but putting it into practice is hard, there's no denying it. But all is not lost because even stress is a habit we can turn around.

Develop the relaxation response

The stress response charges through our body automatically, even a loud bang can set it off. However, we can learn to respond to feelings of stress with relaxation methods to even out our breathing, lower our heart rate and calm our emotions. One simple tip is to take a minute to work through the various muscle groups in your body – tense them really tight for a few seconds and then release, breathing out as you do so. An author I know who is an expert on the subject of emotional healing and who knows a thing or two about how to cope with stress, saw my blog on the 'stomach vacuum' exercise (page 385) and said it was a great way to blow off steam.

Try these on-the-spot relaxation techniques:

- Focus on your breathing for just a couple of minutes. Breathe in for a count of four and out for a count of four, breathing from your tummy. It's easy for our breathing to become shallow when we are stressed or anxious; breathing deeply both calms our mind and gets vital oxygen all around our body, giving us a relaxing boost.
- Go for a five-minute walk. Your stressed mind won't think you can even spare five minutes, but the break will relax you and help you concentrate when you come back to your desk. Likewise, force yourself outside and away from your desk during your lunch break. No one

does useful work while trying to eat and work at the same time, all it does is make you more tired for the afternoon and messes up your digestion.

• Take a couple of minutes to think about the last wonderful, relaxing holiday you were on. Close your eyes and transport yourself there. Feel the sand between your toes, or hear the sounds. Breathe slowly and let your imagination go! Right, I'm off to California . . .

THE RELAXATION DIET

• Asparagus, avocado, leafy greens and oats all contain B vitamins, which are needed to make serotonin, our body's very own good mood chemical.

• Bananas, nuts, chicken and milk all contain tryptophan, which can help with mood and sleep.

• Cucumber is good for a stressed tummy that needs cooling. Or you might need the warmth and comfort of gentle spices like cumin and sweet vegetables like squash and carrots.

• When I am feeling under pressure, I make up a big batch of Congee (see page 33), which is very light on the digestion.

• Berries contain high levels of antioxidants and vitamin C, which can help with stress. If you are stressed, you may notice you are more susceptible to colds and bugs.

Getting a good night's sleep

Sometimes we need energy to get ourselves moving, but when stressed, our minds are often so 'wired' that we can't sleep well and begin to feel frazzled. This is when relaxation techniques can help to calm our body and mind so that we're able to recharge and feel refreshed again. I am very lucky in that it's rare for me not to sleep through the night; my problem is that I struggle to wake up when my vitality is a bit low. But for many, stress equals a poor night's sleep, which only compounds the problem. I have always thought the best advice is to create a relaxing night-time ritual, just as we do for children so that they wind down and automatically know it's time for sleeping. And having a bath in the evening with some relaxing oils like lavender is just about the best tonic for a long and stressful day, even better than a gin and tonic. You might groan, but I'm sure you'll also recognize the fact that alcohol tends to disrupt our sleep, so if you're struggling anyway, then it's a very good idea to replace that with a cup of herbal tea. I like Rooibos in the evening, but whatever takes your fancy and is caffeine-free.

Don't work or surf the web in the couple of hours before you go to bed and you might want to try watching less television. Eat your dinner as early as possible and keep it fairly light so that it's easy on your digestion. And just a few minutes sitting quietly, deep breathing and allowing the stresses and strains of the day to come into your mind and then fade away, can be very helpful in relaxing your body and mind. Lastly, the tip that sleep clinics always give to people is to make sure that your bed is just for sleeping (you don't often hear what they say about sex, but apparently it's helpful too). So it's best to read in the lounge ahead of going to bed and definitely don't have a television or computer in your bedroom if you struggle with insomnia.

Tips for getting a restful night's sleep:

- Wind down before you go to bed
- Avoid caffeine from lunchtime onwards
- Don't eat late
- Don't read, watch TV or work on your laptop in bed
- Try a simple meditation in the evening to begin to quiet your mind
- Drink chamomile tea and have a lavender bath to help you unwind
- Get up early and at the same time every day to help tire you out physically

The power of touch

If you are feeling stressed or anxious, then a good hug or good sex releases a hormone called oxytocin, sometimes called the 'love hormone' because we release it after we have an orgasm. Oxytocin is a feel good hormone, like the endorphins released during exercise. And also, it's good to lean on your friends and loved ones in times of stress as feeling loved and cherished is a scientifically proven antidote to the effects of stress. And yes, it's true, having a pet is just as good because you usually get both healing love and touch as you stroke them.

Dealing with the source of your stress

In *Eat, Pray, Love,* Elizabeth Gilbert recounts the year she got her life back by travelling to Italy, India and Bali. It's one of my favourite books and while not everyone can travel the world to find themselves, it inspires you to take a look at life and rediscover your passions.

When stress gets out of hand, it becomes a passion killer in all senses. A little is good for us, it keeps us on our toes and striving to do well, but we all know that feeling when it changes from a force for action to a knot in the pit of our stomach. I think it's helpful to have a quiet sit down and a think about whether our stress is something we're happy to cope with or if the core source needs addressing. Personally, I don't handle stress brilliantly so I have changed my life to lighten my load. The positive impact on all aspects of life, including my Flat Tummy, have been obvious for all my friends and family to see. Listen to your gut, it's often right! (See Resources for recommended books and websites related to stress.)

How to raise your energy levels

Because some people struggle to relax when stressed, it can be exhausting. To counterbalance the depleting nature of modern-day stressors, these energy-boosting tips are handy to have around as you go through the day. Take your moments to recharge when you can. When it comes to being healthy, if we feel full of vitality and good energy, we tend to gravitate towards healthy foods and enjoy exercise, rather than finding it an impossible 'task'. We have more mental energy to stick to our healthy intentions and are less susceptible to stress and the need for comfort in the form of cake and ice cream. Like everything, it's a question of balance, and we do the best we can.

Water

When we're really busy and feeling a bit under pressure, we often forget to drink much water or take a break for a cup of herbal tea. We get into that mode of thinking that there just aren't enough hours in the day to get everything done, even putting off going to the loo until we're desperate.

Water is a wonderful balancer – when we are hydrated, we simply feel better, but when dehydrated, we feel tense and we might get the stirrings of a headache and then convince ourselves that what we really need is a cup of coffee. Just remember that water nourishes our entire body, from helping our skin to look radiant and younger to aiding our kidneys to perform at their optimum, getting rid of all those modern-day toxins we encounter. Drinking more water also helps with bloating and to keep our appetite in check. Sip room temperature water and warming herbal teas throughout the day.

Beetroot

Healthwise, beetroot is a true super root, known for helping to lower blood pressure. Herbalists call beetroot the 'vitality plant' because it contains antioxidants, magnesium and iron, hardly any fat, very few calories and lots of fibre. Some brave souls drink beetroot juice and if you want the ultimate boost, why not give it a go, but for the mere mortals among us, Beetroot and Apple Soup (see page 273), Beetroot and Feta Couscous (see page 305) or a simple side of roast beetroot, all pack a fantastic nutritional punch.

Grapes

A friend of mine told me the instant snack trick of freezing grapes so they are like mini popsicles, sweet and refreshing. Grapes are high in potassium, so hydrating and detoxing, and they are also high in natural sugar and contain B vitamins that help convert sugar into energy, rather than fat.

Peaches

In China, peaches are associated with immortality, said to revitalize the body and make you more youthful. Peaches are energizing for your skin and, as they contain 80 per cent water and are rich in soluble fibre, they are excellent for keeping you regular, good for your energy levels and your Flat Tummy.

Oats

Oats are the perfect source of complex carbohydrates, which release energy slowly over time rather than giving you a short burst followed by a sharp dip. A great tip is to soften oats overnight in some water and then your morning porridge will take no time to make and be lovely and soft, good for the digestion. When we are feeling stressed, it's easy to rush out of the door in the morning and not have breakfast, especially if our stress is making it difficult to get up on time. Eating a good breakfast is one of the best ways you can ease stress through your diet. It's the time of the day when your digestion is working at its most efficient and sets you up on a positive note, helping you feel balanced and nicely energized, rather than frazzled.

Seaweed

Seaweed never quite made it into the trendy superfood ranks of pomegranate or acai berries and it's not hard to see why. It might not be the prettiest of foods, but seaweed is an underwater gem. For centuries, people all around the British Isles would dry seaweed to provide extra nutrition in the winter. Now we tend to think of Japan when we think of seaweed. The people of Okinawa are known for eating plenty of seaweed and many of them live to 100 and are known for their healthy hearts and low cholesterol levels. Seaweeds contain energy-boosting B vitamins, are good for the brain and skin and strengthen the immune system.

The nice people at Itsu and other sushi cafés get us eating seaweed without even knowing it as lots of sushi is wrapped in seaweed. It's also delicious in miso soup. Nobu do an amazing seaweed salad, but as we can't pop to Nobu every day, try baking strips of the nori seaweed you can now buy in the supermarket and have as a snack.

Sunflower seeds
In Chinese medicine, sunflower seeds are said to be sweet in flavour and that they tonify Qi. Qi is our body's energy and vitality and so foods that are beneficial to Qi are great when we feel in need of a little energy boost. Sunflower seeds are a handy source of vitamin B1, thiamin, which converts blood sugar into energy. So either way you look at it, a handful of sunflower seeds will get you going.

Coconut water
More hydrating than water? Well, that's the claim of this natural, but now very trendy super drink. Coconut water is packed with potassium and is naturally isotonic, helping your body to replenish itself, particularly after exercise.

Green tea
If you fancy a warming energy boost, then you can't beat a pot of freshly made green tea. Green tea has been shown to help lower blood sugar levels and so reduce sweet cravings. Getting our blood sugar nicely balanced is a key to sustained energy, rather than unhelpful highs and lows.

Go for a walk

We often find ourselves sitting for long periods of time, either at work, travelling or relaxing in front of the television. We can literally come to a bit of a grinding halt and one of the best ways to get the energy moving around your body again is to go for a quick walk. If you can pop out for a 15-minute walk at lunchtime rather than working through, you will re-energize for the afternoon ahead and be much more productive than working for that extra time. It's much easier said than always done, don't I know it, but getting into the habit of walking to a particular shop or just going for a meditative wander will refresh both your body and mind.

Natural light

Natural light is energizing for our bodies as it contains vitamin D, which is helpful for our immunity and is a 'good mood' vitamin. During the winter, don't automatically reach for your sunglasses on brighter days – 10 minutes of light without the barrier of glasses is a body and mind tonic.

Ginseng

Ginseng has been shown to help fight off illness, so if you feel a cold coming, add ginseng to your shopping list (along with honey, lemons and thyme for a sore throat). Ginseng is also thought to be beneficial if you are feeling stressed. Stress takes a lot of our energy and so anything we can do to help alleviate stress will also give our energy levels a boost.

Smile

Smile and the world smiles with you. Smiling releases good mood endorphins and it's good for our immune system. Plus it brightens up someone else's day too.

Let go of negative emotions

Now I'm not about to go all woo-woo on you, but I do think it makes sense that holding on to negative emotions takes effort and energy that could be put to far better use elsewhere. Deep-seated emotions are best dealt with by professionals, but the everyday frustrations and sparks of anger or annoyance we all feel are best experienced and then released (gently if possible) so they don't nag away and deplete our energy.

Peppermint, rosemary and ginger essential oils

If you are lacking in energy, then a few drops of one of these essential oils in the bath or mixed with a carrier oil like almond and used for massage, might do the trick. Really good massage therapists will chat to you before your massage and then make up an individual oil based on what you need that day, whether it's energy, calm, creativity or romance.

PLJ

Not a weird tonic, but Pure Lemon Juice. My dad tells me his grandmother had lemon juice and warm water first thing in the morning every day and swore by it. Research does suggest that lemon juice is good for our digestion, and the better our digestion, the better our energy. I am a herbal tea girl in the morning, but have many friends who very happily squeeze a lemon every morning without fail and love the ritual as well as the taste.

Energizing people
Have you noticed how some people give you energy, while others seem to drain it? If you need a boost, then ask your favourite energy-giving friend out for a cup of green tea and a chat.

Have a banana
Still the best-designed snack-on-the-go, despite the mass of cereal bars lining up in the supermarkets. There's also good reason why so many sports people munch on bananas round the golf course or on the tennis court. Bananas give you both a quick and slow releasing burst of energy, plus they are good stress busters and mood improvers (and they are the inspiration for Dawn's Banana Loaf, see page 369).

Natural yoghurt
Ignore all the no-fat, artificially sweetened yoghurts, now practically the whole aisle, and simply choose natural yoghurt for a healthy hit of energizing B vitamins and friendly bacteria. With a drizzle of honey, some fresh berries and nuts or roasted peach, you can't beat it.

Sugar busting
When we want something sweet, we often think of biscuits, cake and milk chocolate first. We think a peach, a pear or a banana just won't cut it, and yet every time we manage to override the hardwiring in our brains, we feel great! I texted a friend to ask for an 'ingredient of the month' and she

replied, 'Peaches. I'm eating one right now and it's so juicy and delicious and everyone else is having jelly babies. They are missing out.'

The key is to have delicious natural alternatives at your fingertips and break the habit of always reaching for chocolate or biscuits, so that you can have them occasionally, but don't need them for a fix. Whenever you can, go for the least processed sugars you can find:

- Berries
- Bananas
- Peaches
- Pears
- Cherries
- Dates
- Figs
- Melon
- Dark chocolate

Green energy
Green leafies are full of energy. Enjoy a cup of nettle tea for a sustaining boost (at the weekend you can even pick your own).

Breathe
It is obvious, but something we often forget, that breathing deeply is the easiest way to access more energy, and it's also calming and helps us think more clearly. Think about it right now. Are you breathing from your tummy as you should be or higher up from your chest, taking shallow, quick breaths? Practise breathing from your tummy at home, in to a count of five and out to a count of five. Keep

your shoulders relaxed and just focus on the breath. Then perhaps when you sit down at your desk or before meetings, take a moment to breathe deeply for a minute or so. A calorie-free instant fix!

KATE'S DAY 15

On rising: Cup of nettle tea
Breakfast: Granola, yoghurt and banana
Snack: ½ Eat Natural bar (yes, half!)
Lunch: Carrot, Ginger and Orange Soup (see page 75)
Snack: Clementine
Dinner: Vegetarian Chilli (see page 338) with a dollop of
    Greek yoghurt, strip of dark chocolate
Drinks: 3 x cups of green tea, 5 x glasses of water

Exercise: Tae Bo workout

Tip of the day Drinking lots of water and herbal tea is a
simple trick for getting a flatter tummy, but isn't always easy
or desirable! Buy a lovely jug to fill with water and keep on
your desk. If you are at home, a good filter system is a good
idea, and every time you have a spare moment, pop the
kettle on, take a minute to breathe deeply and slowly and
make yourself a cup of herbal tea.

YOUR DAY 15

On rising:
....

Breakfast:
....

....

Snack:
....

Lunch:
....

....

Snack:
....

Dinner:
....

....

Drinks:
....

Exercise:
....

KATE'S DAY 16

On rising: Cup of green tea
Breakfast: Granola with raspberries and yoghurt
Snack: Miso soup
Lunch: Green salad, monkfish, fennel and broccoli (out
   to lunch)
Snack: Innocent superfood smoothie
Dinner: Carrot, Ginger and Orange Soup (see page 275),
   2 seeded oatcakes, strip of dark chocolate
Drinks: 3 x cups of green tea, 4 x glasses of water, fresh
   mint tea

Exercise: 12,000 steps, 10 minutes of Flat Tummy
   Workout (see page 377)

Tip of the day If you prefer savoury to sweet, then a cup of
miso soup late morning is fantastic for seeing you through to
lunch with hardly any calories and lots of nutrition. It comes
in very handy sachets and I drink mine from a Japanese-style
bowl cup, though a mug will do!

YOUR DAY 16

On rising:
....

Breakfast:
....

....

Snack:
....

Lunch:
....

....

Snack:
....

Dinner:
....

....

Drinks:
....

Exercise:
....

KATE'S DAY 17

On rising: Cup of dandelion tea

Breakfast: Omelette with mushrooms (see page 309)

Snack: Clementine

Lunch: Carrot and coriander soup and flatbread

Snack: Banana

Dinner: Lemon and Ginger Salmon (see page 313) with pak choy and spring onions, natural yoghurt with honey, ½ strip of dark chocolate

Drinks: 3 x cups of green tea, 1 x cup of nettle tea, 3 x glasses of water, decaf coffee (I thought I'd best go for decaf as caffeine might have a strong effect on me by now)

Exercise: 18,000 steps, 10 minutes of Flat Tummy Workout (see page 377)

Tip of the day If you prefer sweet to savoury, then finding delicious ways to add more fruit to your day will smooth your path to a flatter tummy. Buy a big bag of cherries for everyone at work to share – it seems to add to their appeal. Make a simple fruit salad of berries, banana and pear with a lovely squeeze of lemon juice over the top. Chop up fresh pineapples, mango or melon in the morning and take to work in your trusty Tupperware.

YOUR DAY 17

On rising:
....

Breakfast:
....

....

Snack:
....

Lunch:
....

....

Snack:
....

Dinner:
....

....

Drinks:
....

Exercise:
....

KATE'S DAY 18

On rising: Lemon juice and hot water

Breakfast: Porridge with Quick-and-Easy Berry Compote (see page 264)

Snack: Pear

Lunch: Tapas – chickèn, lamb, hummus, pitta bread, cheese pastry, artichoke, courgette

Snack: Slice of melon

Dinner: Beetroot and Apple Soup (see page 273), yoghurt

Drinks: 3 x cups of herbal tea, 1 x glass of spicy tomato juice, 3 x glasses of water

Exercise: 14,000 steps, 10 minutes of Flat Tummy Workout (see page 377)

Tip of the day Spicy tomato juice is the perfect alternative to a glass of wine if you are out for lunch.

YOUR DAY 18

On rising:
....

Breakfast:
....

....

Snack:
....

Lunch:
....

....

Snack:
....

Dinner:
....

....

Drinks:
....

Exercise:
....

rising: Cup of green tea

reakfast: Porridge

Snack: Banana

Lunch: Leek and potato soup with wheat-free bread

Snack: Pear

Dinner: Tuna Stir-Fry (see page 318), strip of dark
chocolate

Drinks: Lots of herbal tea and water during the day

Exercise: 12,000 steps, 10 minutes of Flat Tummy
Workout (see page 377)

Tip of the day A healthy breakfast is essential for healthy
weight loss.

YOUR DAY 19

On rising:
....

Breakfast:
....
....

Snack:
....

Lunch:
....
....

Snack:
....

Dinner:
....
....

Drinks:
....

Exercise:
....

KATE'S DAY 20

On rising: Cup of nettle tea
Breakfast: Porridge with hazelnuts, cinnamon and honey
Snack: Eat Natural bar
Lunch: A whole avocado and beetroot soup
Snack: Banana
Dinner: Veggie Crumble (see page 340)
Drinks: 6 x cups of herbal tea

Exercise: 10-mile walk

Tip of the day Remember that if you do an intensive work-out, go for a long walk or run in a day, then you'll be able to eat more and still lose weight. If you've had a busy day at work and exercise is impossible, then you need to be aware of this. Keep your meals and snacks on the lighter side, but still eat regularly throughout the day to keep your blood sugar nicely balanced.

YOUR DAY 20

On rising:
....

Breakfast:
....

....

Snack:
....

Lunch:
....

....

Snack:
....

Dinner:
....

....

Drinks:
....

Exercise:
....

KATE'S DAY 21

On rising: Cup of green tea
Breakfast: Scrambled eggs with mushrooms
Snack: Banana
Lunch: Superfood Salad (see page 292)
Dinner: Rest of the Veggie Crumble, natural yoghurt with
a little honey, ½ strip of dark chocolate
Drinks: 6 x cups of herbal tea

Exercise: 10,000 steps, 10 minutes of Flat Tummy
Workout (see page 377)

Tip of the day Don't go hungry or your healthy intentions
will go out of the window.

KATE'S DAY 21

On rising:
....

Breakfast:
....

....

Snack:
....

Lunch:
....

....

Snack:
....

Dinner:
....

....

Drinks:
....

Exercise:
....

5
Maintenance

Keeping on the Straight and Narrow-waisted

When I lost weight I had both a specific goal and a more general aim. Initially, I had six weeks until I was leaving my then current job and going off on a round-the-world trip. New Zealand and California both featured prominently on my itinerary and I wanted to regain both my body confidence for the beaches and my energy for making the most of the trip and all the wonderful places I would be visiting. And my long-term goal was to get back to the balanced style of healthy living that had gradually gone by the wayside over the past few years – I might never be a health nut, but I wanted to tip things back into my favour.

I lost just over a stone before my holiday and did worry that I might ruin all my hard work with a couple of months of eating and drinking my way around the world. But the strong foundations had been carefully laid, almost without my realizing it, and I lost another half stone while I was away. Because my energy levels were so much better, I walked and walked wherever I could, from the suburbs of

Tokyo to the beaches of Los Angeles. I enjoyed almost everything I ate and must admit I savoured a glass of wine with most of my meals, but I also looked at all the menus to find local, fresh dishes. My green tea habit stayed with me throughout the trip to balance out the morning cup of coffee and I sought out food markets wherever I could for the colours, smells and inspiration.

Once I was back home, I discovered the one key to keeping to my healthy intentions was to enjoy them. The rest of my excess weight gradually disappeared – I had reached my own goal of losing 1 ½ stone, so the extra ½ stone was a bonus. I'll be honest, I don't make myself a freshly squeezed juice every morning because I can't face the nightmare of washing up a juicer. But my porridge habit has stuck firm and it's still my breakfast of choice most days. And once a week or more, I'll wander along to the grocer's with the specific aim of gathering soup ingredients, even if it's just the simplest of combinations – carrot, onion and ginger.

Firing up your passion for food and your interest in all things healthy is a great ally. I'd never been a vegetable lover before, but by learning about seasonality and asking everyone I know for delicious ways to cook with them, I have had a genuine change of heart. While on a visit to my parents in Dorset, they introduced to me to the wonder that is their local organic farm shop. I thought my senses had gone haywire as the colours and textures of all the vegetables were so vivid and so fresh. I took a bag of brightly coloured chard home and it looked so inviting all chopped up in the colander. It tasted just as good and my parents have been seeing a lot more of me as I now come back with a bag of inspiring seasonal veg every time I visit. This is what the Flat Tummy Club is all about.

And I've even gone along to exercise classes with friends for the first time in my life, proving it's never too late to try new things.

How to Keep Going Until You Reach Your Goal

- You should be in a rhythm after the first three weeks of buying and cooking healthy foods, exercising and side-stepping challenges.
- Keep up your diary if you want to, but once you are confident your healthy habits are ingrained, then just use it for the odd note and some planning.
- If you need to lose quite a bit of weight over time, like I did, then don't feel you can't ever enjoy a celebration or treat, but also remember that your appetite and taste buds are changing, so go for a smaller piece of cake or one scone instead of two.
- Don't think of the weekends as opportunities to binge while you punish yourself during the week – keep to a happy and healthy balance throughout the week.
- Continue to weigh yourself once a week to check your progress and tweak your diet or exercise to keep things on a gentle downward curve.
- Try the Weekend Detox (see page 226) if you ever need a burst of health to keep you going.
- You do have to keep thinking and choosing carefully while you lose weight, but I think of this as being self-aware rather than constantly telling myself 'no'. I don't want to go back to my old eating and drinking habits because I felt rubbish back then.
- The more exercise you can fit in, the easier it will be to reach your goal.

- Stick to eating natural, whole foods wherever possible and your body will find its healthy weight.
- Always have a healthy breakfast.
- Eat plenty of soup and pack in those fruits and vegetables.
- As my very slim friend says, 'Never go hungry,' so always make sure you have a plentiful supply of healthy snacks.

The Weight Loss Plateau

It's natural to entertain discouraging thoughts if you hit a weight loss plateau before you reach your end goal, but I've come to realize that for me, the periods of time when I stayed the same weight for a while broke up the whole process into natural stages.

Lots of books tell you to immediately make your portions smaller or shun all carbohydrates to trigger continued weight loss. But I think because I took a more long-term view to wanting a healthy lifestyle, I was able to relax when I hit a plateau and take the time to realize I'd made a brilliant effort to get there, not beat myself over the head. When I was ready, I would then tweak my diet and exercise to drop a few more pounds. I have no scientific evidence to back this up, but if I ever felt anxious about how my weight loss was going, as soon as I lightened up, relaxed and reminded myself to simply enjoy everything I ate and did and to follow my own body intuition that had developed over the months, I seemed to miraculously drop a couple of pounds.

How to Maintain Your Weight Loss

Once you reach your goal – ta da – the advice remains pretty similar as I hope you will have made some lifelong lifestyle changes.

- Continue to weigh yourself once a week, just to keep a gentle eye on your weight.
- Don't let your healthy lifestyle fall down your list of priorities – keep remembering all the positive effects it has on all aspects of your life.
- Enjoy occasional splurges, don't feel guilty about them and don't get attached to them.
- If you feel yourself slipping back into old habits, then keep a food diary for a few days and you will soon see what you need to tweak to get back in balance. For me, I still have to keep an eye out or I will fall back into the habit of pouring a glass of wine every evening.
- Don't binge at the weekend. Focus on keeping a healthy balance whatever the day of the week and if you are ever in need of a burst of healthy living, try the Weekend Detox (see page 226).
- Keep engaging your brain to think about what you eat. You have developed the self awareness to know what's good for your body and what to avoid.
- Keep cooking.
- Discover your local farmer's market, grocer or farm shop and experiment with new ingredients and flavours.
- Ask your friends if they'd like to try a new exercise class with you.
- If you go through a very stressful time in life and struggle to keep to your healthy habits, then don't feel

guilty, but do look after yourself and deal with stress rather than letting it build and build (see page 179).
- Keep up your relaxation techniques and healthy rituals.

Tales from the Club
I got it into my head after having my third baby that I had to go on a strict raw food diet to get back in shape. But then you reminded me that I had simply eaten healthily when trying to conceive and that I really enjoyed healthy food. I also worried about whether I could still eat too much, whether it was chocolate or vegetables, and you said just relax, there was little chance of eating too many vegetables! So once I did relax and started my gentle Pilates every week (see page 243 for Flat Tummy Mummy), I realized that soon I was back in balance and it's a place I am very happy to be!

Healthy Holidays

(Or . . . No More Wind Beneath Your Wings)

My mum came up with that alternative title for this chapter and laughed at her own joke for about an hour and a half. But as she says, wind is a very common side effect of travelling, especially on long haul-flights, and it's not much fun spending the first few days of your holiday feeling bloated and uncomfortable.

Travelling is a Flat Tummy challenge that uses boredom and desperation as its allies to break us down. When you're on a train journey, the clinking of bottles and wheels that signify the near arrival of the trolley is a moment of tremendous excitement when you've been staring out of the window for the past half hour, lulled by the movement into a stupor. You watch the trolley make its way towards you, trying to catch a glimpse of what's on offer. And then you realize *there's nothing good on the trolley*. Your healthy option is a bottle of water, what a treat. And yet it's so tempting to have something just to keep you occupied for a while.

It's the same on long-haul flights. The best feature of the

dinner service is that it passes a bit of time, although unfortunately, not as much as you'd like as the cabin crew always seem to want to serve drinks, get the trays out and clear up in world record time, leaving another eight hours stretched out ahead for you to regret eating that pudding so fast, well, eating that pudding full stop.

I think the term 'mindless eating' perfectly suits how we tend to eat while travelling. I was driving back to London one day and stopped at a service station for a quick break as the roads were busy. All I wanted was a cup of coffee, but then there was this big sign that declared I could order a chocolate muffin to go with my coffee for only 10 pence more than the coffee alone. I didn't stop to think, I ordered the deal and ate the whole muffin, all the time thinking, 'I don't even like this, it's full of rubbish, why am I eating it?'

Now when I'm travelling, I think about when I'll be on the train or plane or need a break from driving and organize myself so that I won't have to resort to nasty cheap flight paninis or giant packets of crisps from the trolley. I went on holiday with friends to Spain and arrived a bit later on a different flight. My friends asked if I wanted dinner and I replied that I'd made myself a little picnic for the flight. It was a little thing, but they were so jealous of my simple ham roll and a banana, which were easy on the tummy and meant I arrived feeling great, rather than with that all too familiar bloaty feeling.

While I was losing weight, I went on a round the world trip. This involved quite a few long-haul flights and the last thing I wanted to do was to eat rubbish or get terrible wind for days at a time, so I prepared my hand luggage for my healthy holidays. Here's what you do.

Snacks and Teas

- Herbal teas are the perfect way to take in more fluid during flying without the caffeine that comes with the standard tea and coffee options. You might wonder if it's even possible to ask for anything other than tea or coffee, but the crew can always bring you a cup of hot water, as I've discovered. Teas that are particularly calming for the tummy include chamomile, peppermint and linden flowers. My favourite is jasmine tea as it just instantly relaxes me.
- Bananas
- Apples
- Oranges (these also smell lovely and refreshing as you peel them)
- Eat Natural bars
- Trail mix
- Dark chocolate (instead of the nasty dessert on the tray with a cup of gut rot coffee, enjoy a cup of herbal tea with a piece of your own chocolate)
- Oatcakes (my favourite varieties are cheese, fruit, dark chocolate or ginger and come in handy snack packs)
- Ricola (this is a bit random, but I do like to have the odd sweet to suck while travelling and these contain more natural ingredients than many boiled sweets)

Tips for the Journey

- Instead of a double gin and tonic, start your flight with a spicy tomato juice. I never drink this at home, but it's the perfect in-flight drink. Orange juice can be a bit acidic and anything carbonated will sit in your stomach as you sit cramped in your chair, not a good combination. You instantly feel you are making a healthy choice and this tends to have a positive impact on the rest of your flight.

- Don't feel you have to eat at the pace of everyone else around you. I don't know why people eat so fast when they have hours of flight ahead. Take your time. Even though it's not the most delicious food you've tasted, chew each mouthful and put down your cutlery in between.

- Don't feel you have to eat everything that's put in front of you. The dessert and rectangle of plastic cheese will call out to you, but if you have your own little stash of healthy alternatives, you can stay strong.

- Before your return flight, seek out a few local snacks for the journey. I will often take a freshly made roll and some fruit with me and not bother with the airplane food at all.

- Drink plenty of water during the flight and don't worry if it means you have to keep waking up the person next to you to get to the loo. It's much better to get up regularly, both for your circulation and for your digestion.

Tips for Your Holiday

Don't get me wrong, holidays are for treats and having a great time, whether you love to chill out with a book and a cocktail by the pool, spend a week camping and cooking sausages on the gas stove in the countryside or go on a culinary and cultural expedition. Holidays are also the perfect time to really enjoy being healthy – so that we come back revitalized and keen to keep that energized feeling.

- Ask in restaurants for the local, seasonal specialities. These will often be the freshest, healthiest ingredients.
- If you are by the beach or pool, then swimming is great exercise and invigorating. If you're camping or on a city break, then you'll likely find you do lots of walking. Again, this is really healthy for balancing out the treats.
- Start the day with fresh fruit.
- Treat yourself to a spa treatment or take some lovely spa products with you.
- Give yourself 10 minutes a day for a mini yoga, Flat Tummy Workout (see page 377) or Pilates programme.
- Chill out and unwind. Our stressful lives so often lead to putting healthy living on the backburner. This is the perfect time to bring it back to the forefront.
- Have a big salad as a starter with just a simple dressing of a little oil and the local vinegar.
- Go for a stroll after dinner.
- Nourish your mind with books and culture. Thinking make us healthy.
- Share dessert!

Viva Flat Tummy Club!
There were the odd instances while on holiday in Spain last week when my friends placed a knowing question mark at the end of 'The Flat Tummy Club'? When I come across a local speciality, like the freshly cooked churros (doughnuts) and chocolate dipping sauce, then I'm going to try them! But that's the beauty of Flat Tummy Club

– my friend and I shared the doughnuts and then, an hour later, we were having an equally great time scouring the town market for juicy pears, peaches, grapes and melon, which Natalie turned into the most delicious fruit salad. I also had my birthday on holiday and as I tend to put my cooking feet up when I go away, my friends created an amazing birthday dinner of red snapper, giant prawns and a tortilla to die for.

So we've had lots of treats, but we've also been walking or jogging in the mornings, swimming, devouring tomatoes and even did some tummy exercises on the balcony! Plus Natalie is going home reinvigorated about jogging and determined to give up Coca Cola when she's back at work and Dawn is saying goodbye to biscuits. A healthy, balanced holiday . . .

Here are Dawn and Natalie's delicious holiday recipes:

Natalie's very easy baked snapper

Fillet the fish (or ask your fishmonger to do this for you) and smother with olive oil, mixed herbs and fresh rosemary. Stuff with sliced garlic and lemon slices and season with salt and pepper. Cover with tin foil and bake for 15 minutes on a medium heat. Serve with a salad.

Dawn's lemon, rosemary and balsamic chicken

Mix up a marinade of olive oil, fresh rosemary, the juice of half a lemon juice and a sliced garlic clove (optional) and put your chicken breasts in the marinade for, say, 20 minutes. Heat a frying pan and then place the chicken on the hot pan. Cook for about 5 minutes on each side, depending on the size of the breast (if you flatten the chicken breast, it will cook much quicker). Add a dessertspoon of good balsamic vinegar 2 minutes from the end of the cooking process and cover the pan with a plate or some foil. Serve with something that makes your tummy flat.

Et voilà!

Out to Dinner

There is a restaurant I go to fairly regularly that serves the best Eggs Benedict with the best home fries in London. I'm happy to splurge on Eggs Benedict once in a while now I've lost weight, but of course I gave them a wide berth initially. I remember going to the restaurant and as I sat down, I was panicking inside – would I want to eat anything else? And if I did, would I be really disappointed? Well, it was a revelation. I enjoyed scouring the menu for the freshest, most delicious looking alternative I could find and settled on the sea bass, which was absolutely mouthwatering. I ate every morsel and felt just that right kind of satisfied, rather than overfull. I won't be so angelic every time, but it's good to know I can be!

Here are some general tips for eating out, and then a few specifics for certain types of cuisine:

- Don't arrive starving hungry so that you devour the bread basket.
- A friend of mine orders water and a little jug of fresh lime juice to mix with it; it's lovely and refreshing if you find water boring.

- Take your time and focus on the menu, rather than chatting merrily away and then having to decide on the spot when the waiter arrives.
- Go for lots of fresh vegetable sides and steer clear of side dishes like honeyed parsnips. In a lot of restaurants, this will mean more honey than parsnip.
- I often start with a simple rocket and Parmesan salad.
- Fish is usually a great choice and often something you might not make at home.
- For lunch, two starters and lots of vegetables can work really well.
- Initially while you are losing weight, steer clear of dessert and as a general rule, if you really fancy it, then share, as usually a couple of mouthfuls are all you need to round off a nice meal.
- Fresh mint tea or green tea is lovely to end a meal with.

Italian

In Italy, pasta and risotto dishes are usually served as starter sizes rather than main courses, which is a good rule of thumb to follow. The Italians do beautiful vegetable dishes and tomato salads, fish and chicken. They use olive oil, lemon juice and lots of wonderful herbs, all of which are healthy ingredients and why the Mediterranean diet it heralded as one of the best. Even a glass of red wine is thought to be good for us. I don't want to put a dampener on things, but watch out for all the olive oil as it's still very rich and best in small quantities. The dessert tiramisu is one of my favourite things in the world and I don't even have a very sweet tooth, so if I'm going to a great Italian restaurant, I'll make sure to have a big walk beforehand!

Indian

Many of the dishes we are used to ordering in our local Indian are quite rich and creamy, especially korma and chicken tikka masala. Be adventurous and try more regional dishes from the menu. The chicken tikka that comes out sizzling on the skillet is a great choice as it has fantastic flavour without a rich sauce. Order plenty of vegetable dishes and share your mains and rice. Likewise, if there are a few of you, share a naan bread rather than having one each, or be strong and say no thank you.

Chinese

The traditional Chinese diet is full of vegetables, soups and amazing flavours. Unfortunately, the dishes in our local takeaway are often very sweet, sticky and full of MSG. I find MSG makes me feel weird, so I tend to avoid restaurants that use it in their cooking. Look for soup-based dishes, vegetable dishes and avoid anything deep-fried. Swap fried rice for steamed rice or a simple noodle dish.

Japanese

Japanese is a great healthy option, from sushi to miso soups to delicate aromatic flavours. I remember wandering in to a tiny restaurant in Tokyo by the side of a little old railway station and being served the most delicious set lunch. The Japanese do this so well – the tray they give you is an art form in itself with miniature dishes of pickles, a cup of miso broth, a few mouthfuls of the most amazing seaweed salad and then the main dish, often pork or tofu with steamed rice. It was fresh, yet warming and comforting at the same time away from the chilly spring day. Jasmine tea was topped up in a beautiful little ceramic cup throughout and everyone chatted quietly. It was the most serene experience, the complete opposite to a bustling trattoria in Rome, but good for the digestion!

Thai

Thai flavour combinations are also full of healthy ingredients, from coconut to lime, ginger to lemongrass and Thai basil. Fish, prawns and vegetables are abundant in Thai cooking and I also find that portions are usually pretty perfect in Thai restaurants, not too big, but always satisfying.

Traditional British

Seasonal British cooking is becoming increasingly popular, especially with the rise of the gastro pub. The only problem is that whenever I go out for a weekend lunch in the pub, I feel stuffed – portions of meat are often twice what you'd have at home, potatoes are roasted in duck fat, chips are twice-fried, fish is covered in butter or batter. I'm all for a treat, but sometimes I find it just too much. My sister loves a carvery, though, and her tips for avoiding a total blowout are to just have one or two small potatoes, go for the leanest meat and lots of vegetables.

Weekend Detox

Sometimes the thought of a detox is almost luxurious as it signals a retreat and a bit of time for ourself. Occasionally, I like to turn the concept of what I consider to be treats on its head. After all, if the most expensive destination spas in the world can feed you broth and make you feel like your body is a temple again, then I'm sure we can manage it at home.

Some nutritionists are extremely keen on either 'going raw' or even fasting over a weekend. I've never managed this, so I've put together my own version of a weekend detox, still very healthy and wholesome, but which doesn't lead to me escaping my own personal 'fat farm' for a quick pint in the pub.

You might want to start your Flat Tummy Club plan with the weekend detox, but don't feel obliged if it's too much of a sudden change. I do the odd detox when I can detect that I may be just at the start of a slippery slope back into bad habits.

For Starters

The key to a weekend detox is a balance of rest, relax-ation and a bit of activity for both your body and mind.

We tend to put quite a lot of strain on our digestion in normal modern life and on our stress levels, each feeding the other. I'm not hardcore about this, but I also think we are somewhat surrounded by chemicals and toxins, especially if we live in a city. We lurch from pristine, chemical-clean environments to hot, stuffy buses and tube trains, with goodness knows how many germs passing among us. A cleansing weekend is a chance to enjoy the simpler things in life and give our bodies a bit of nurturing.

The basics of a weekend detox include:

- A 12-hour break overnight between dinner and breakfast (i.e. an early dinner)
- Keeping food choices easy on the digestion
- Supporting your liver
- Supporting elimination (yes, bowel movements)
- Calming and refreshing your mind
- Gentle exercise

COLONIC REVIEW (ANON, UNDERSTANDABLY)

The main point I can remember is that it's pretty EXPENSIVE! A fantastic woman called Sue made me feel like it was just the most natural thing in the world to be discussing books with a plastic tube in a place where really there shouldn't be a plastic tube. I did it after I'd been on a diet for three months. I was determined to return to a less harsh eating regime, but to stay really healthy and it seemed like an appropriate 'kick start'. I had two, two weeks apart, with a course of charcoal tablets in between, which 'stick' to all the bad stuff. The second one is REALLY cleansing – I felt fantastic afterwards, incredibly flat in the stomach department and 'light'. My skin was amazing and I didn't want to eat anything but organic veg and brown rice! Sue said I'd know when I needed to come back and she was absolutely right. I think everyone should try it once, and it's not nearly as embarrassing as you might think, or maybe that's just age . . .

Detox Recipes

DETOX SMOOTHIE

Honeydew melon, peeled, deseeded and chopped
Frozen seedless grapes
¼ cucumber, peeled, deseeded and chopped
Weak jasmine tea, chilled

Put everything in a blender and whizz it all up.

DESERT ISLAND DETOX SMOOTHIE

½ frozen banana
Small cup of fresh pineapple
50ml coconut water
1 tablespoon natural yoghurt

Put everything in a blender and whizz it all up, adding water until you get the desired consistency.

QUINOA AND CINNAMON PORRIDGE

If you want to simply make oat porridge, then go ahead, but you might fancy trying quinoa as an alternative while you are having such a healthy and interesting weekend! The great thing is that you can cook a load of plain quinoa and keep it in the fridge for a few days. Then you just have to heat it up and add bits and bobs as you like, whether for breakfast or supper. You can add a dash of milk with some honey and a sprinkle of cinnamon, dried cranberries or raisins and almond flakes. If you want to avoid dairy, then add a little almond or hazelnut milk instead.

NETTLES

In *Hatfield's Herbal*, Gabrielle Hatfield describes nettle as vigorous and one of nature's great survivors. And interestingly, its uses by modern-day herbalists still reflect those qualities. I have often been recommended to drink nettle tea because it is considered fortifying and a general tonic. In Chinese medicine, they use the term 'blood nourishing' to describe nettle broth or tea, and when you think that it is full of iron, that makes sense. Like dandelion, nettles are also diuretic, so are cleansing, great when you are making gentle and healthy changes to your diet. It can take a little time to acquire the taste for both of these herbal teas, but once you do, they are wonderfully comforting and, yes, nourishing. In the spring especially, you can make nettle tea yourself with the young nettle tops (about the top half dozen leaves on the plant). It does make me laugh, popping out to the garden with gloves on to gather nettle leaves, but I also enjoy the ritual of making a pot of fresh tea. And if you suffer from hay fever, then make fresh nettle tea as soon as the young plants grow and keep drinking through the spring to help prevent the onset.

NETTLE BROTH (FROM *HATFIELD'S HERBAL*)

Gather plenty of fresh, young clean nettle tops. Soften chopped onions in a saucepan with a little olive oil over a moderate heat, add chopped carrots and continue to soften. Add chicken stock and the rinsed, chopped nettle tops and simmer for around 20 minutes until tender, seasoning to taste.

MISO SOUP WITH ALL THE TRIMMINGS

SERVES TWO
About an inch of fresh ginger, finely sliced
2 tablespoons miso paste
2 spring onions, finely sliced
1 green chilli, finely sliced (optional)
1 head of pak choy, roughly chopped
A handful of bean sprouts
Splash of mirin
Splash of wheat-free tamari sauce (Japanese soy sauce)

1. Bring 500ml water to the boil and add half the ginger. Simmer for a couple of minutes.
2. Dissolve the miso paste in half a cup full of the hot water, then add to the pan and stir so that it all dissolves.
3. Add the spring onion, chilli, pak choy and bean sprouts and simmer gently for a few minutes.

4. Add a splash of mirin and tamari to taste, and the rest of the ginger before serving.

LEMON AND GINGER BARLEY WATER

This will probably remind you of when you were poorly as a child. Well, your mum was right. Lemon barley water is fortifying and refreshing. Lemons are the perfect detox ingredient – squeeze into hot water for your first drink of the day and make a simple dressing with extra-virgin olive oil for salads and veggies.

MAKES JUST UNDER A LITRE
50g pearl barley
Zest and juice of 2 unwaxed lemons
½ teaspoon grated fresh ginger
2 tablespoons honey, or to taste

1. Put the pearl barley, lemon zest, ginger and 1 litre water into a pan. Bring to the boil and simmer for 10 minutes.
2. Strain into a bowl and add the honey and lemon juice.
3. Leave to cool.

POACHED SALMON AND WATERCRESS

Salmon and watercress are the perfect healthy partners. Salmon contains lots of essential fats, while watercress has been described as a great hangover cure. Irish monks called it a 'pure' food and apparently Hippocrates chose the site for his first hospital by a stream so that he could grow fresh watercress for his patients. It's also packed with vitamin C and nutrients that may help the liver and immune system.

1. Simply poach your salmon fillet in enough water to cover with a good sprig of dill. Bring the water to the boil, add the salmon and dill and simmer gently for about 10 minutes until the salmon is cooked through.
2. Serve with watercress and a dressing of lemon juice, a little apple cider vinegar and lots of freshly ground black pepper.

ENERGY SALAD

Cruciferous vegetables are full of nutrients that are healthy in just about every way possible for food! They have anti-cancer properties, help to keep your heart healthy and generally boost your vitality.

To assemble an energy salad, simply chop up ultra fresh and crunchy cabbage, fennel and carrot very fine, sprinkle with sesame seeds and squeeze over lemon juice and a little hazelnut oil. Vitality on a plate!

RICE WITH SESAME AND GINGER VEGETABLES

Now, if you want to have simple brown rice here, then go for it – it's unrefined and definitely high in fibre. I'm also going to introduce you to something the author Emma Cannon introduced me to, called congee. Emma is an acupuncturist who specializes in women's health and she gave me an article on congee, I tried it that very same evening and have been addicted ever since.

For anyone with digestive weakness, congee is something of a revelation. In Chinese medicine, the digestion is the foundation of health and, in particular, our 'spleen energy'. If you ever feel that your thoughts or feelings are spilling over and affecting how well your tummy feels, then this is because your spleen energy is depleted. Many of us feel like this every once in a while, or even quite often if we are natural worriers, so taking time out over the weekend and eating simple and nourishing food is the perfect way to get back on track. The spleen also appreciates touch, like massage or even a nice hug, and because it's what gives us a sense of belonging in our own body, it's also closely connected with nature. Perhaps that's why destination spas and our own home-made detox weekends tend to feel even better with a combination of fresh foods, pampering and relaxation in our surroundings.

Congee is very simply polished white rice (not brown or basmati) cooked in lots of liquid for a long time, literally until it's completely broken down. I was extremely suspicious before making it that it would be, well, awful, but I have to admit to exclaiming out loud after the first mouthful just how delicious it was! It is extremely gentle on the tummy and very versatile because you can add savoury or sweet toppings.

CONGEE

PER PERSON
40-50g rice
Vegetable or chicken stock (optional)

1. Simply rinse the rice until the water comes through clear. Add to a pan along with about 7 times the amount of water. If you are having savoury congee, you can add a little vegetable or chicken stock to the water for extra flavour.
2. Bring the water to the boil and then reduce to a very low simmer, leaving uncovered.
3. You can stir the rice once it starts getting thick to stop it

sticking to the bottom. It doesn't matter that you break up the rice, as it will do that anyway.

4. Once the rice looks like glue or gloop, about an hour to an hour and a half, it's ready. It looks like it will taste of pure starch, but you will be very pleasantly surprised, I promise.

5. One of the simplest things to serve with your congee is aromatic vegetables. I will often steam some tenderstem or purple sprouting broccoli and add to the bowl with shards of fresh ginger, scatter over some pumpkin seeds and drizzle with sesame oil and soy sauce. To add protein to the dish, I stir-fry some chicken.

Home Spa

Body brushing

Body or 'skin' brushing is something you can do at home every day to help stimulate your circulation. We excrete and eliminate waste products through our skin, just as our liver and kidneys are also organs of elimination.

Body brushing has been around in various forms for centuries. The Comanche Indians were known to scrub their bodies with sand from the Texas River; the Japanese would traditionally brush with a loofah before taking a hot bath; and in Russia, *platza* is a traditional skin brushing with a *venik* made of a bundle of oak or birch leaves after a bath. The *venik* can be soaked in olive oil, which also combines with the natural oils of the leaves on warm skin, opening and cleansing the pores, while the brushing action stimulates the circulation and metabolism.

Body brushing is also thought to support the lymph system that, like the bloodstream, goes all around our bodies, but instead of carrying blood, carries a clear liquid high in white blood cells called lymph. The lymph system is a major filtering system for the body and also helps us to fight infections as part of the immune system.

How to body brush

- Do this before your shower on dry skin.
- Use a natural bristled brush, ideally with a long handle so you can reach your back.
- Don't brush your face or anywhere that feels tender. Women shouldn't brush their breasts. Start with gentle brushing for the first few days.
- It's best to skin brush for a couple of minutes before your shower.
- Always brush towards your heart.
- Start with the soles of your feet and up each leg.
- Brush from the hands along your arms to your shoulders.
- Brush upwards on the buttocks and lower back.
- Use a gentle motion on the abdomen towards the centre.
- Brush from the back of the neck to the front and gently on the chest towards the heart (just to repeat, but not on the breasts).

Note: if you have any medical condition, then check with your doctor first.

Home-made body scrub
Instead of putting sugar in your tea, here is a simple recipe for making your own spa body scrub. Use any essential oils you like. Lavender is relaxing, grapefruit and ginger

energizing and coconut simply makes you feel like you're on holiday.

- Pour some light brown demerara sugar into a bowl. Add some rock salt or coarse sea salt.
- Add half almond oil, half honey to fully cover the sugar/salt.
- Add a few drops of essential oil.

I am always on the lookout for healthy tips to share for the Flat Tummy Club and this journey often means finding things from around the world or back in the past. I remember going through some old boxes of memorabilia my dad had kept after his parents passed away. He pulled out a little pamphlet put together during the war by a hospital association, full of fantastic and simple health advice. I loved a particular article titled 'Pep up that Circulation' by Jean Forbes:

The secret of looking warm and beautiful in spite of icy weather and fuel rationing can be given in one sentence – pep up your circulation . . .

So that you start the day warm, do a few arm-swinging exercises when you jump out of bed, and just watch how this brings the blood to the face, replacing the pinched look with a rosy glow. Touch your toes 20 times . . .

Exercises over, sponge yourself down with lukewarm water, gradually lowering the temperature as the days pass till you are using water that is quite cold. Follow this by a rub-a-dub-dub with a rough towel. Don't stop when you are dry, but starting from the ankles give yourself a second rubbing and scrub the limbs towards the heart . . .

Have something hot with your breakfast – porridge is grand . . . walk a short part of the way to work. Step out briskly, breathing deeply and rhythmically as you walk. Breathe in to a count of eight steps, and then let your breath out slowly to another count of eight. Try it! Before you've gone spanking along for five minutes, your eyes will be sparkling, your cheeks glowing, and you'll feel on top of the world.

Exercise

As Jean said in the 1940s, a brisk walk is perfect. Taking a bit of time to do some floor stretches, yoga or Pilates is also just right for a cleansing weekend. You might want to avoid going to the gym or out for a hard run as these are quite intense, but each to their own.

Meditation

Inner Space in Covent Garden, London, has a fantastic website with guided meditations and also provides free meditation workshops in its centre (see Resources). If you have never tried meditation, then I can't recommend these highly enough. The online meditations are just a couple of minutes each, but have a deeply relaxing and positive effect on me every time.

Here are some pointers they give to go alongside the meditations:

- Make an appointment with yourself for 10 or 20 minutes each morning or evening
- Find a quiet place and relax
- Sit comfortably, upright on the floor or in a chair
- Keep your eyes open and, without staring, gently rest them on a chosen point somewhere in front of you in the room
- Gently withdraw your attention from all sights and sounds
- Allow your thoughts to follow a guided meditation
- Don't try to stop thinking – just be the observer
- Gradually your thoughts will slow down and you will begin to feel more peaceful
- Acknowledge and appreciate the positive feelings and thoughts that may spring directly from the meditation
- Be stable in these feelings for a few minutes
- Finish your meditation by closing your eyes for a few moments and creating complete silence in your mind

A Schedule for Unwinding

As soon as you wake up, get up

On rising: Sit quietly with a cup of lemon juice and hot water, nettle or dandelion tea

Meditate for 10 minutes or so

Body brushing and a lovely shower with a natural body scrub

Flat Tummy Workout (see page 377) or some yoga if you prefer

Breakfast: Quinoa and Cinnamon Porridge (see page 229)

After breakfast: Go for a good walk and take a banana and a flask of green tea

Lunch: Energy Salad (see page 232)
Chill out for the afternoon, reading or listening to music
Make a lovely fruit salad

Early dinner: Congee (see page 233)

Before bedtime: 10 minutes meditation

Drinks: Plenty of water and/or herbal teas throughout the day

IMMUNE BOOSTERS

If you ever feel the start of a cold or sore throat, or you want to help your body ward off bugs over the winter months, then nature provides some helpful immune boosters that are well worth giving a try:

• No surprises here, but the more fruit and veg you can cram into your day, then the more immune-boosting vitamins you will take on board, especially vitamin C. And I've learnt that taking a big load of vitamin C all in one go isn't such a great idea because you won't absorb it all and it'll just go straight through you. Berries are particularly good, as are green leafy vegetables.

- Clipper Tea do a very tasty green tea with echinacea, the perfect combination for the colder months as green tea helps with weight loss while echinacea will help in warding off colds.
- Vitamin E helps too, and can be found in nuts and seeds and olive oil.
- Get some omega-3 fatty acids into your weekly diet with oily fish, walnuts, olive oil and kidney beans, which are all good sources.
- Probiotics can be good, so natural yoghurts are a great idea.
- Where you can, add garlic to your recipes. Garlic and onions are great natural flu fighters.
- Crussh do a lovely 'flu fighter' made with apple, pear, lemon and ginger. You can also try making your own at home by warming honey, lemon juice, crushed ginger, water and, if you are brave, some garlic and cayenne pepper for extra strength.
- Thyme-infused honey is great for a sore throat.
- Comfort yourself with Portuguese Chicken and Mint Soup (see page 278). Not only is it comforting, but intensely nourishing and easy to digest. The perfect recuperation food.

For Her

Many women find that they put on weight more easily over the years and also find it tough to get back in shape after having children. Even our monthly periods can cause our weight to fluctuate quite dramatically and trigger cravings for more sugary foods, or simply more food full stop. I have included just some introductory ideas here as any of these subjects are complex enough for their own books.

PMS

We need a chapter on 'What to eat when your period starts'. My carrot and coriander soup and Terrance [sic] Stamp bread only got me as far as 4.30 and then I ate my boss's leftover Pret Carrot Cake.

I had a look into this. It's not the case for every woman, but over half of us experience food cravings at some point in the run up to our period and it'll be no surprise that it is down to hormones. As oestrogen levels go up and down, so does the stress hormone cortisol. When cortisol is high enough, it triggers our body to go into fight or flight mode and stimulates appetite to feed that fight or flight. But we don't actually need to fight or flee, so we just put a few extra pounds on! Plus serotonin – the good mood hormone – often goes down about now so we crave carbs to get a quick mood fix. We tend to fall into two camps – sweet or savoury – but in both cases it's a combination of fats and carbs that we crave – so things like buttery toast, crisps and cheese for the savouries and chocolate, ice cream and cakes for the sweets.

So, what can we do about it? It seems the crucial thing is to make sure you eat more coming up to your period, but fill up on complex carbs so that you don't reach for the quick fixes. Essential fatty acids are also really helpful in balancing out those blood sugar spikes. Refined sugars really do just make it worse, and steer clear of caffeine and alcohol around this time as the key is to stay in balance, not have huge ups and downs.

Eat more . . .
Salmon
Avocado
Wholegrains
Chicken
Almonds
Asparagus
Berries

Drink more . . .
Water (for the dreaded PMS bloating too)
Herbal teas (nettle, dandelion and ginger are all great)

Other tips for PMS

- Eat little and often to keep your blood sugar in balance, rather than big meals with nothing in-between.
- Some won't like me much for saying this, but exercise helps balance those stressed-out hormones and stop you going into fight or flight mode.
- Stress doesn't help, so it's a good time of the month to go for a massage, have lovely aromatherapy baths, early nights and try relaxation techniques (see page 237).

Flat Tummy Mummy

I've included a section devoted to mums because it's something I am asked about more than anything else. I've got together with top Pilates coach Elanor Wallis–Scott and everyone I know who has had children to create a mini guide.

The first thing to say is obvious, but not always so easy in this modern world – to be kind to yourself and take your recovery after having a baby very gently. I realize that's not what we see in the glossy magazines every month, but your health and wellbeing are too important to sacrifice for the sake of a bit of extra time.

Recent studies have shown that unfortunately many women feel that postnatal support and information is not quite as comprehensive as they would hope for, often due to a simple lack of time and resources. Do feel that you can ask anything you want, like when you can start to exercise again and what exact exercises are right for you, as this will depend on the type of birth and how your body is recovering. Most women who have had a caesarean, for example, will be advised not to start exercising or lifting until at least six weeks after the birth and no one should start any kind of exercise without the all clear from her doctor. Often you can be referred to a physiotherapist to show you the core exercises that will gently start to strengthen your abdomen muscles and, of course, your pelvic floor.

What happens to your tummy during and after pregnancy?

To state the blindingly obvious, your tummy has to do a lot of expanding during pregnancy. The joints and ligaments are made more supple by hormones that allow give in the pelvis and abdomen to accommodate your growing baby and in preparation for birth.

After pregnancy, women are often left with weak abdominal muscles and softness in the pelvic floor. Strain in the lower back through pregnancy can also continue because the abdomen and pelvis are a key source of support for the back and posture.

Diastasis recti

Think of your abdominal muscles as a corset that wraps around your middle. During pregnancy, that corset loosens itself from the front and, for about two thirds of women, creates a gap between your muscles called *diastasis recti*. This is where there is a separation between the left and right side of the rectus abdominis muscle that covers the front of the tummy – the 'six pack'. The key question is just how much of a gap and also whether your muscles naturally return in the months after giving birth or need a bit of extra help.

Measuring the gap

To find out how big the gap is between your recti muscles, you simply lie down on your back with a small pillow to support your head. As you do a gentle crunch (but don't just lift your head off the floor, engage your abdomen), you can feel with your fingers for your 'sixpack' muscles and whether you can fit your fingers in the gap in the middle. One or two fingers width is normal after pregnancy, any more than that and you need to be careful when it comes to doing abdominal exercises. Do ask your doctor if you aren't sure. Many women aren't even aware of this condition and end up doing exercises like crunches and obliques that make it worse, not better. The key is to bring the muscles back together before you then start to strengthen them.

Elanor's Pilates workout for mums

With all cases, I start with pelvic floor exercises and deep abdominal work, working from the inside out as you begin to remember where your muscles are.

Pelvic floor

Start by sitting on a chair (I find the chair helps you to feel what you're meant to be doing). Think about lifting the vaginal outlet up towards the centre of the body (imagine you're drawing water up a straw). You'll only be able to lift a little bit to begin with, but slowly the muscle will get stronger. The aim is to gradually lift for longer and longer until you can do so for 5 breaths.

You will need to get all outlets strong and as we have three, we've got work to do. Again, start by sitting on a chair, hands resting on your legs, and lift up your urethra outlet, then release; lift up your vaginal outlet, then release; lift up your rectal outlet, then release. Then go back to the vagina and urethra and start all over again. At first it'll be slow and a bit clumsy, but persevere and you'll become a dab hand. These are great to do on the bus, train, supermarket queue and even during a boring conversation.

Pelvic floor and deep abdominal
Your body has been through a lot during pregnancy and birth. You need to give it time. I usually tell my new mothers that it'll take the body at least the same amount of time to mend as it took to grow the baby – so absolutely no pressure. These exercises are fantastic for gently aiding the body on its road to recovery.

- Lie on your back with your knees bent, feet on the floor. The feet, knees, hips and shoulders should be in line with each other and the head in the middle of the shoulders. This is the semi-supine position.
- Put your hands on the area between your naval and pubic bone, keeping all your joints relaxed. Take a breath in through the nose and as you blow the air out on a long stream of breath, sink your lower abdominals (the area between your naval and your pubic bone) down towards your spine. You should feel your deep abdominal wall tightening. Think of a corset being tightened around you.
- When you breathe in again release the abdominal wall and start again.

When you have mastered the exercise above, add the following: As you breathe out and deepen your abdominal wall towards your spine, at the same time draw your pelvic floor muscles up. The muscle fibres of the deep abdominal wall are mixed with the muscle fibres of the pelvic floor, so when one gets activated, the other one gets activated too. It's great to become aware of this physically and to strengthen them in unison.

Diastasis recti exercise
Start in the same position as above, but this time wrap your arms around your abdominals.

- Breathe in and then, as you breathe out, lower the deep abdominals towards your spine, tilt your pelvis underneath you and draw your hands towards each other, putting slight pressure on the two sides of the rectus abdominis muscle (six pack) towards the middle (imagining your muscles knitting back together). Breathe in to recover and on the outward breath, start again.
- Repeat for 5 minutes.

Shoulders
I remember feeding at night and getting a really sore neck and shoulders, so here are some gentle exercises to open up the chest and upper spine and ease the neck.

- Fold a large bath towel lengthways and then roll it to create a roll. It shouldn't be too fat
- Lie on your back with your knees bent, feet on floor. Place the towel either on or just beneath your shoulder blades, interlock your fingers behind your head and allow your upper spine to relax over the towel.
- Hold this for 3 breaths. Repeat for 5.

- Place the towel lengthways along your spine, so that it supports your bottom all the way to your head. Take your arms out to the side with the palms facing up towards the ceiling. Keep the knees bent and the feet firmly planted into the floor. This is also great for opening up the chest and softening the spine.
- In a sitting position, place your hands on your shoulders and circle your elbows around, 5 in one direction, 5 in the other.
- To help a sore neck, turn your head from side to side, making the movements slow and small.

Cat stretch

The main aim of this exercise is to increase spinal articulation.

- On your hands and knees, breathe in and, as you breathe out, curve your spine into an angry cat position. Hold this position as you breathe in again, and then uncurl your spine as you breathe out.
- Repeat for 5.

Pelvic circles

On your hands and knees, keep your spine relaxed as you make circular movements with your pelvis. This is great for warming up and releasing the pelvic region.

Bridge

- Lie on your back with your knees bent, feet on the floor. The feet, knees, hips and shoulders should be in line with each other and the head in the middle of the shoulders.

- Breathe in and, as you breathe out, tilt your pelvis under, peeling each vertebra from the floor one at a time. You will end up resting on your thoracic vertebrae (just below the shoulder blades).
- Breathe in as you hold this position and, as you breathe out, lower the spine, one bone at a time, back to the starting position. Keep your feet well planted on the floor throughout.
- Repeat 4 times.

Abdominal lift (not to be done if there is diastasis recti)
- Lie on your back with your knees bent, feet on the floor. The feet, knees, hips and shoulders should be in line with each other and the head in the middle of the shoulders.
- Interlock your hands behind your head. Breathe in and, as you breathe out, lift your head and chest and slide the ribs towards the pelvis
- Keep the pelvis heavy and breathe in to hold. Lower back to the start position as you breathe out.
- Repeat 6 times.

Oblique (not to be done if there is diastasis recti)
- Lie on your back with your knees bent, feet on the floor. The feet, knees, hips and shoulders should be in line with each other and the head in the middle of the shoulders.
- Begin by placing your right hand behind your head and your left hand by your right leg. Breathe in and, as you breathe out, rotate your left side towards your right, allowing your arm to follow. Breathe in and hold and, as you breathe out, lower back to the start position.
- Repeat on the other side. Do 3 on each side.

Gentle hip rolls

- Lie on your back with your knees bent, feet on the floor. The feet, knees, hips and shoulders should be in line with each other and the head in the middle of the shoulders.
- Bring your knees together and take your arms out to the side with your palms facing down. Breathe in and, as you breathe out, take your knees over to one side, keep your feet together, and roll your head over in the opposite direction.
- Breathe to hold and then return to the start on the outward breath.
- Repeat 3 times on each side.

Lifting and baby carriers

You'll do plenty of lifting as a mum – I was always very impressed at how my mum could out-carry my dad when it came to shopping (or was it a ruse?). My friend says her arms have never been more toned, but she definitely has to stop and think more about her tummy muscles and her back when she's picking up her toddler or carrying her baby in a sling. The same rules for everyone apply with lifting, but it's just worth repeating because you have to do so much of it. Engage your core tummy muscles as you lift and bend at the knees to come down to what or who you are lifting, rather than bending from the back.

When you are carrying your baby in a sling, keep your shoulders down and straight as they might have a tendency to either tense up or curl forward. Again, keep your core engaged as you walk and you'll get the perfect workout while helping your baby to nod off.

Plenty of nourishing food

I'm the last person who wants to take away your Cadbury's Dairy Milk – it seems like the least you deserve. All I'll say is that when you're ready, I suspect you'll know exactly which foods you need to replace more often than not with some healthy alternatives. You've read all about healthy eating for your pregnancy and this is the perfect time to create a healthy balanced lifestyle for your whole family.

- You might need to wean yourself off the slightly bigger portions that you would've been used to in the last few months of pregnancy.
- I've got some friends who developed a passion for rubbish chocolate during pregnancy and it's not surprisingly a habit that's hard to kick when you're sleeping in fits and starts during the night, giving feeds every couple of hours and generally feeling shattered. Have plenty of comfort foods like soups and stews and maybe, if you eat lots of vegetables, it will pay dividends when your baby grows up and eats her greens!
- Have a good breakfast even if you feel done in from the night before – porridge is very comforting.
- If you have more than one child, then try not to eat the remains of their tea.

Snacks

I've included a list of snacks on page 119 and mums need these more than anyone to keep your energy nicely balanced through the day (well, in an ideal world). Nairn's oat biscuits come in very handy snack packs, bananas and clementines come in their own biodegradable wrappers and see if you can wean yourself off milk chocolate and onto dark. If you can get out for a good long walk, then Eat Natural bars are perfect.

Planning

Once you have a family, I think your powers of planning develop exponentially out of sheer necessity. When they are little, it revolves around food, activities and naps and it doesn't change all that much until they leave for college. So make your healthy life part of the weekly plan, whether it's getting outside every day at some point for a half hour walk, working out your meals for the week so that you can double up some days and then just reheat the next, or perhaps finding out if there is a mother and baby yoga class in your area.

The Menopause – Before, During and After

Hormonal changes during the menopause do lead women to tend to put on some weight. If this is evenly distributed and just a few pounds, then it's actually thought to help reduce the risk of osteoporosis. So if you have gone up from a size 10 to 12, then you are probably eating really healthily. However, many women tend to put on quite a bit of weight around their upper abdomen and, unfortunately, this is the type of fat associated with an increased risk of heart disease.

I spoke to my mum about this time of life and we realized that while there are countless books to guide you through the menopause, there is very little for afterwards. Mum says this just about sums up how many women can feel on occasion, 'Well, that's it then'. You start to feel a bit frumpy and don't really know what to wear anymore, you're not sure your husband cares that much either about how you look and you give in more to temptations because you feel, after all this time, you deserve it. But it's not all negative – you also realize it's a time of life for renewal and doing the things you love: being creative, travelling, making new friends. You might have a little more time to take care of your health and you certainly don't take it for granted any more.

Both my sister and I, in our thirties, are amazed by the energy of our parents' generation – they always seem to be up to something. And it's really this spirit that you need to channel into healthy living. My dad does volunteer weeding at the local farm once a week – he gets a workout, interesting chat and a free bag of organic veggies all at the same time, which balances out all the puddings at the golf club! Mum has always loved yoga and since making a few little changes courtesy of Flat Tummy Club, I've seen a renewed sense of energy. If there is a promise of an egg and bacon bap at the start of it, mum will even join me for two hours of cliff walking along the Dorset coast.

A nutritionist I know who embodies the combination of healthy living with healthy attitude most is Suzi Grant. Suzi is 60 and, as she says, she doesn't expect to look like she did in her thirties, 'but I do expect to *feel* like I did: full of life, enthusiasm, energy, vitality and glowing with health'.

Healthy body

- Apples, rice and yams are often recommended for the post-menopause as these foods contain natural oestrogen
- Gentle exercise like yoga is brilliant for body and mind, flexibility and strength

- Try to reduce your portions a touch as your body is burning off the calories at a slightly slower rate over time
- Walk wherever, whenever you can

Healthy mind

- Deal with stress (see page 179)
- Keep setting mini goals
- Try new things
- Keep your mind active, even after retirement
- Go for lots of haircuts and massages

For Him

By their late 30s, men start to lose muscle strength and it gets harder to stay in shape. Your metabolism begins to slow down, which isn't a bad thing in itself as a high metabolism would put too much pressure on your body as you get a bit older, but it does mean that you need less fuel to keep going. The trouble is that many men grow up being able to eat whatever they like, knowing they will just burn it all off. By the time the correlation between what you eat and the size of your tummy starts to show, it's really difficult to simply eat less.

The Beer Belly

Does it really exist? The annoying answer is yes *and* no, because men who drink more tend to put on more weight, but it is not specifically related to the belly area, which has a lot more to do with genetics.

However, many men tend to put weight on around their tummies more than, say, their bums and thighs, so if you drink too much beer, or eat too much food, it still ends up on the belly. It makes it a simple, if not all that appealing equation:

Drink Less = Lose Belly

Easier said than done?

When I lost my excess weight, I decided to give up alcohol for at least the first two weeks, to help my willpower when it came to food and to prove to myself that I could live without that glass of wine at the end of the day. Because I was on a mission, it wasn't too bad, although I did have a bath most evenings to distract myself.

We all know drinking too much is bad for us, but are we being truly honest with ourselves, especially when it comes to working out how many units we might drink in an average week? A pint of beer, that's about a unit, right? The same for a glass of wine? A pint of 5% beer is 3 units and a glass of 12% wine is 2, that's my weekly unit count doubled in an instant.

Diaries at the ready . . .

I think a drinking diary is even harder to be honest about than a food diary, but once you see the reality in black and white, it definitely helps with your resolve. If you have a smartphone, the NHS has created a free app for counting your daily and weekly units (see Resources), but a good old notebook and pen will also do the trick, and you could photocopy the table on page 257 and stick it in the front for reference.

I know a few men who have given up drinking for a month or two and while they don't go into ecstatic detail about it, the general consensus is that it's not as hard as you think, you'll sleep much better and generally have a lot more energy. One man I know didn't even let it affect his social life in the slightest. He went out, sang karaoke and danced, all without the aid of booze. He didn't stay out quite so late, but his wife was so thrilled that turned out to be a good thing too.

Drink	Average Alcohol %	Volume	Units
Red wine	13%	Standard 175ml glass	2.28
White wine	12%	Large 250ml glass	3
Ale	4%	Pint	2.27
Lager	5%	330ml bottle	1.65
Cider	5%	Pint	2.84
Vodka	40%	Single 25ml shot	1

Source: *www.drinkaware.co.uk*

More Flat Tummy Tips for Men

- Exercising as part of your commute means that you can stay fit while often saving money and time. A friend of mine takes a 'Boris Bike' from Waterloo to the City every day; he doesn't need to change because the bikes only go at a decent potter and now gets 2 ½ hours extra exercise a week.
- Working lunches often mean lots of rich foods and wine but go for two starters and extra veg instead and you'll feel much better for the rest of the day.
- Football with the kids; get out in the garden and go for it.

- Big Daddy portions aren't always necessary. The key is to take your time eating and try putting a little less on your plate just to see.
- Get out in the garden and you can get fit while also growing your own food. And lots of men I know are really getting into cooking, the more you cook the more you'll know what you need to do to flatten that belly.
- Just as many men suffer from bloating as women, the main causes include swallowing too much air by eating too fast or chewing gum, constipation from eating too little fibre, not exercising enough or not drinking enough fluids, or gas-forming foods like beans and cabbage. Good tips include not adding lots of fibre too quickly to your diet but introducing these foods gradually, steer clear of beer (what a surprise) and drink plenty of water and herbal teas during the day.

6

Flat Tummy Recipes

I am not the world's greatest cook, but I have found that developing a growing passion for healthy cooking and ingredients has been great both for my figure and for my general sense of wellbeing. When I first started my plan, ditching ready meals and processed foods was high on my list of actions, so I cooked easy meals that never made me feel like I was on some kind of weird diet or that I was denying myself. If you love to cook, then use this to your advantage and challenge yourself to find and create your own delicious healthy meals. If, as I was, you are a bit of a novice in the kitchen, then be not afraid; if I can make it, then anyone can.

I truly recommend making your own soups as a way to get started and also to explore the fantastic variety of natural ingredients we have at our fingertips. Take the humble carrot; in soup form it goes brilliantly with ginger, orange or coriander, and that's just for starters.

I don't have an internal calorie counter, but I have included calories counts for the following recipes just to give an idea of the types of recipes that are super slimming and others that are perfect after a long day's walking or once you reach your healthy weight and want to stay there. The principles behind the recipes are incredibly simple – they steer clear of lots of starchy or refined carbohydrates, avoid high doses of cream, butter and cheese and include lean proteins, lots of vegetables, herbs, spices and a sprinkling of whole grains. Just a simple, healthy mix of natural ingredients.

Cook's Notes

Unless otherwise specified, all eggs are medium and milk is semi-skimmed. In recipes which include stock I have not added extra salt as shop-bought stock is usually salty enough.

Quick Ticks ✓

I have highlighted any recipes that take less than 30 minutes to prepare, and I do mean take a normal human being less than 30 minutes!

Nutritional Information

Included after many recipes in this section is a nutritional breakdown. It shows the calories, protein, carbohydrate, total fat, saturated fat, fibre, sugar, and salt content of one portion. Not included in the analysis are optional items or serving suggestions.

Breakfast

All the clichés are true: a good breakfast sets you up for the day, gives your brain as well as your body energy, and all those slow-releasing sugars help to keep you well and truly away from the biscuit tin. A Flat Tummy Club member used to skip breakfast, but eat a packet of Mini Cheddars if she had a morning meeting just to stop her tummy rumbling. Now she enjoys a big breakfast of fruit and yoghurt or porridge every day without fail and hasn't looked back.

I have included portion sizes in the list of ideas for breakfast below, just so you can check at the start if your idea of a healthy portion is about right or needs tweaking. Once you see it in the bowl, you can then do it by eye.

A Few Quick Ideas

40g porridge oats with about 150ml semi-skimmed milk (rest water) with 1 tablespoon honey soft prunes, or Quick-and-Easy Berry Compote (see page 264)

40g muesli (or pop to a good health food shop and gather the ingredients to make your own) with about 150ml semi-skimmed milk

20g granola, as many berries as you like and a small pot of natural yoghurt

Fresh mango with a tablespoon of warm Quick-and-Easy Berry Compote (see page 254) and a heaped tablespoon (about 30g) 2% Greek yoghurt

Sliced pear and banana with a squeeze of lemon or lime juice and small pot of natural yoghurt

Drizzle some honey (about a teaspoon) over a halved grapefruit in the evening and by the morning the honey will have softened the sharpness of the grapefruit. Enjoy with a pot of yoghurt and sprinkle (20g) of granola over the top

You can also make porridge with quinoa instead of oats for a change (see page 229)

I've recently discovered nut milks. They're really nice as well as being low in calories and containing no added sugar, so they make a great alternative to milk in your porridge

Weekend Brunches

Grilled mushrooms and tomatoes on a slice of seeded toast

Scrambled eggs (2) and a little smoked salmon (50g) on a slice of toasted soda bread

Poached eggs (2) on toasted soda bread (2 slices)

Grilled lean back bacon (2 slices) and mushrooms on a slice of toasted walnut bread

BREAKFAST MUFFINS

My friend Dawn adapted a recipe from Jo Pratt's *In the Mood for Food* and I can personally recommend these warm with just a little butter on a Sunday morning.

MAKES NINE MUFFINS
175g wholemeal self-raising flour
2 teaspoons baking powder
5 tablespoons wheatbran
2 tablespoons linseeds
3 tablespoons sunflower seeds
1 tablespoons pumpkin seeds
Grated zest of 1 orange
50g dried blueberries
3 tablespoons groundnut oil
75ml agave syrup or honey
2 large eggs
250ml low-fat natural yoghurt

1. Preheat the oven to 190°C/375°F/gas 5. Line a muffin tin with nine cases.
2. Stir together the flour, baking powder, wheatbran, linseeds, sunflower seeds, pumpkin seeds, orange zest and blueberries.
3. Add the oil, agave syrup, eggs and yoghurt and mix until just combined.
4. Spoon into the cases and bake in the oven for between 20 to 25 minutes. Cool slightly before serving.

Nutrition per portion: 211 kcal, protein 8g, carbohydrate 27g, fat 9g, saturated fat 1.7g, fibre 4.2g, sugar 12.6g, salt 0.53g

✓ QUICK-AND-EASY BERRY COMPOTE

When berries are in season and you can go gathering, then you'll be lucky enough to make this with fruit straight from the bushes, but equally in the cold winter months, using frozen fruit to make warm compote is an easy way to add wonderful flavour to porridge or yoghurt.

MAKES ABOUT A JAM JAR'S FULL (3–4 PORTIONS)

Simply put a punnet of frozen mixed berries into a pan with a few squeezes of agave syrup or honey and a little water and warm over a gentle heat until the fruit starts to break up. Taste to check the sweetness. Enjoy immediately or leave to cool and then transfer to a jam jar or container and store in the fridge for a few days.

Nutrition per portion: 39 kcal, protein 0.75g, carbohydrate 9g, fat 0.25g, saturated fat 0g, fibre 2.38g, sugar 9.1g, salt 0.03g

✓ FLAT TUMMY CLUB BERRY SMOOTHIE

This is the easiest smoothie to make and it's simply delicious. It gets you off to a quick start with your five-a-day
and the lemon juice gets your digestion going, while the
yoghurt is satisfying protein and full of friendly bacteria.

PER PERSON
A couple of handfuls of frozen mixed berries
½ banana
2 heaped tablespoons natural yoghurt
Squeeze of fresh lemon juice
Fresh apple juice, as needed for consistency

Put everything in a blender and whizz it all up.

Nutrition per portion: 183 kcal, protein 5g, carbohydrate 38g, fat 2g,
saturated fat 1g, fibre 4.7g, sugar 37.1g, salt 0.15g

✓ FANTASTIC FRESHLY SQUEEZED JUICE COMBINATIONS

I do not juice at home because of the washing up involved, but if I had a personal juice chef, I'd have one every day as my mid-morning snack!

Carrot, apple and ginger
Carrot and orange
Carrot and blackberry
Pineapple, pear and ginger
Apple, melon and mint
Apple, kiwi and lime
Apple, cucumber and celery
Apple, pineapple and watermelon
Beetroot, pear and lime (not for the faint hearted!)

Soups

I am evangelical about soups when it comes to weight loss, flat tummies and wellbeing in general. A simple bowl of soup is something that cultures from all corners of the world share in common. There's a good reason why we crave chicken soup when we are ill – it's so easy to digest and packed with natural goodness.

The really good news about soup is that research tells us that per calorie, soup is more filling than other foods like, say, a sandwich. And if, like me, you struggle to eat your five-a-day, then a bowl of vegetable soup usually provides at least two portions.

The International Language of Soup

As a health publisher I have been introduced to traditional medicine practices from many cultures, including Chinese medicine and Indian Ayurveda. Soups are prominent in both these traditions and in particular kitchari in Ayurveda and congee (see page 233) in Chinese medicine are rice soups that are both considered excellent for digestive health. The Chinese will often have a broth or soup with every meal, even breakfast.

On your travels, you will always discover a new soup if you ask for the local speciality. There is a little bakery café in Tavira, Portugal, where I first discovered Portuguese Chicken and Mint Soup (see page 278). It cost a euro and was divine. A friend of mine often makes Vietnamese Pho (see page 284) and, while visiting Mauritius with a Mauritian friend, I remember vividly her cousin telling us about 'Magic Soup', which women will eat after pregnancy both because it is so nourishing, but also because it helps them to regain their figures. It's simply vegetable soup made with whatever is to hand, but what a great name.

For the ultimate combinations, steer clear of potato or pasta-based soups while you are losing weight. Personally, I don't find rice bloating and for me it turns soup into a main meal, but as ever, listen to your body and how you react to different foods.

While losing the weight, have a BIG soup or salad every day for lunch or dinner whenever possible. Even better, I remember that in American cafés (of the healthy variety) you can often order a cup of soup and a small salad – perfect. If you have bread, then go for flatbreads or sourdough. Make loads of soup at the weekend and you can store instant meals for the week ahead.

Simple Stocks

For me, stock tends to come in a tub with the word 'bouillon' on the side. But my Flat Tummy friends who make their own stock, especially chicken, rave about the difference between home-made and shop bought. You can certainly control the amount of salt you use when making your own stock and it's good to keep in mind that many shop-bought stocks are quite high in salt, so don't add any more to your soups and stews (remember, salt encourages our body to retain water, not very helpful for a Flat Tummy). Home-made stocks also transform simple recipes into delicious dishes.

VEGETABLE STOCK

MAKES ABOUT 2 LITRES STOCK
2 onions
1 leek
2 carrots
2 sticks of celery
1 fennel bulb or a parsnip
1 bay leaf
1 teaspoon black peppercorns
½ teaspoon coarse sea salt

1. Chop all the vegetable into big pieces and add to a large saucepan along with all the other ingredients. Fill the pan with water.
2. Bring to the boil and then lower to a gentle simmer for up to 2 hours. Add more water along the way if needed.
3. Allow to cool and sieve into containers. Freeze until needed.

CHICKEN STOCK

MAKES ABOUT 3 LITRES STOCK
1 whole organic/free-range uncooked chicken
75g fresh ginger, peeled and cut into strips
5 fat cloves of garlic, unpeeled
1 carrot, peeled and roughly chopped
1 leek, roughly chopped
1 onion, roughly chopped
1 stick of celery, roughly chopped
1 bay leaf
1 teaspoon black peppercorns
½ teaspoon coarse sea salt

1. Place the chicken in a large saucepan. Cover with 3.5 litres water, then add all the other ingredients.
2. Bring to the boil, skim and then reduce to a gentle simmer for up to 6 hours, skimming off the fat with a slotted spoon ever so often. You can add more water during the process.
3. Strain the stock through a fine sieve and save the best bits of chicken to use for soup.
4. Allow to cool and then freeze in batches.

CELERIAC, WILD MUSHROOM AND ROSEMARY SOUP

Hugo Shuttleworth, who owns Berwyn Catering and Events, is a healthy chef I know and so this soup is a bit special, but definitely worth all the ingredients.

SERVES THREE TO FOUR
10g dried porcini or chanterelle mushrooms
2 rashers of pancetta, chopped (optional)
1 tablespoon olive oil
2 large banana shallots (or 5 small ones), finely chopped
1 clove of garlic, finely chopped
400g peeled celeriac, chopped into large chunks
2 tablespoons vermouth (such as Noilly Prat) or white wine
500ml chicken (or vegetable) stock
1 bay leaf
1 sprig of rosemary

1. In a bowl, pour hot water on to the dried mushrooms and leave to soak for 15 minutes.
2. Fry the pancetta in the olive oil over a medium heat until it is translucent and has released most of its fat, then add the shallots, lower the heat and cover the pan.
3. When the shallots have softened for about 5 minutes, drain the mushrooms (reserving the mushroom-flavoured soaking water), chop them finely and add to the shallots. Raise the heat slightly, fry for a couple of minutes, then add the garlic and the celeriac. Stir everything well and leave to cook for a couple of minutes before adding the vermouth. Let the vermouth cook down for a minute or so, then add the stock, mushroom soaking liquid (beware grit!) and the herbs.
4. Bring the pan to a simmer and leave it gently cooking for

about 20 minutes, by which time the celeriac should be very soft. Remove the herbs, season and liquidize. Season to taste. For a creamier texture, pass the soup through a fine sieve.

Nutrition per portion: 90 kcal, protein 3g, carbohydrate 7g, fat 5g, saturated fat 0.5g, fibre 6.3g, sugar 4g, salt 1.59g

BEETROOT AND APPLE SOUP

Beetroot is an acquired taste, but just one look at this soup
and you can feel the healthy powers. Beetroot is said to be
cleansing and good for the liver, perfect for when your diet
needs a bit of a tidy up.

SERVES THREE TO FOUR
1 tablespoon olive oil
1 onion, chopped
3 raw medium beetroots, peeled and chopped
Sprig of fresh thyme
500ml vegetable stock
1 big eating apple, peeled, cored and chopped

1. Soften the onion gently in the olive oil or butter so that
   it is translucent, not browned.
2. Add the beetroot, thyme and stock and simmer for about
   10 minutes.
3. Add the apple and simmer for another 5 minutes or so.
4. Blitz everything in a blender and season to taste. I add a
   spoonful of 2% Greek yoghurt if to hand.

Nutrition per portion: 113 kcal, protein 2g, carbohydrate 17g, fat 5g,
saturated fat 0.5g, fibre 3.2g, sugar 14g, salt 1.84g

✓ BUTTERNUT SQUASH AND PEAR SOUP

Pear adds a lovely subtle sweetness to this autumnal soup, so if you are craving comfort, then make up a batch rather than reaching for the cakes. Orange-coloured vegetables contain beta-carotene, a natural antioxidant, and while they might not be quite so super as the green leafies, they add vibrancy to our diet.

SERVES THREE TO FOUR
1 onion, sliced
1 tablespoon olive oil
1 stick of celery, chopped
1 medium butternut squash, peeled and roughly chopped
500ml vegetable stock
1 pear, peeled, cored and chopped

1. Soften the onion in the olive oil over a low heat for 5 minutes. Add the celery and soften for a few more minutes.
2. When translucent, add the butternut squash and, after a minute or so, add enough stock to cover the vegetables.
3. Simmer for 5 minutes, add the pear and then simmer until the squash is easy to pierce with a fork, about another 5 minutes, but this will depend on your squash.
4. Blitz in a blender and check the seasoning before serving.

Nutrition per portion: 181 kcal, protein 4g, carbohydrate 33g, fat 5g, saturated fat 0.5g, fibre 6.1g, sugar 20.1g, salt 1.75g

✓ CARROT, GINGER AND ORANGE SOUP

A melody of orange in this soup, with a gentle healthy kick from the ginger. This soup packs a vitamin C punch, while ginger is warming and great for the digestion.

SERVES THREE TO FOUR
1 tablespoon olive oil
1 onion, finely chopped
1 stick of celery, finely chopped
3 or 4 carrots, peeled and chopped
½ teaspoon grated fresh ginger
500ml vegetable stock
A juicy orange, peeled

1. Gently soften the onion in the olive oil over a low heat for 5 minutes, add the celery and continue to soften for a few more minutes.
2. Add the carrot and ginger, give everything a good stir and cook for a minute or so before pouring over enough vegetable stock to cover the vegetables. Simmer for about 10 minutes until the carrot is soft enough to pierce with a fork.
3. Squeeze and break up the peeled orange, almost crumbling it into the pan, but leaving out any tough pith.
4. Purée in a blender in batches and check the seasoning.

Nutrition per portion: 112 kcal, protein 2g, carbohydrate 16g, fat 5g, saturated fat 0.6g, fibre 3.9g, sugar 13.9g, salt 1.78g

GAZPACHO

This is a summer spectacular of a soup from Hen. Cucumber is great for water retention; onion is up on the list of top healthy foods, along with garlic; there's MUFAs in the form of olive oil and even a little vinegar, which is thought to help the body absorb nutrients. You can also add extras to the soup once made, which helps make it more sustaining. I like chopped-up egg, cucumber, green pepper and ham. Also, if you want to leave out the bread from the soup, I don't think that matters, it just makes for a slightly thinner soup.

SERVES FOUR
6 or 7 tomatoes
1 green or red pepper, deseeded and roughly chopped
1 cucumber, peeled and chopped
1 onion, chopped
2 or 3 slices of slightly stale bread, crusts removed and broken into small pieces
2 tablespoons red wine vinegar
Sea salt and freshly ground black pepper
1 or 2 cloves of garlic, crushed
2 tablespoons olive oil

1. With a knife, take out the green eye of the tomatoes and place in a bowl. Pour over boiling water and leave for 30 seconds. Run under cold water, peel away the skins and chop.
2. Put all of the vegetables in a deep bowl with the bread and mix together thoroughly.
3. Add the vinegar, 600ml water, salt, pepper and garlic.
4. Pour into a blender, half at a time, and purée for about 1 minute until smooth.

5. Put the purée into a bowl and gradually beat in the olive oil using a whisk.
6. Cover lightly and refrigerate until thoroughly chilled.
7. Before serving, whisk the soup to ensure that all the ingredients are blended.

Nutrition per portion: 134 kcal, protein 4g, carbohydrate 16g, fat 6g, saturated fat 0.9g, fibre 3.1g, sugar 8.2g, salt 0.69g

PORTUGUESE CHICKEN AND MINT SOUP

An FTC member wrote a very nice review for this warming soup:

> *This is one of those 'too good to be true' recipes –*
> *it's so simple, uses very few ingredients and yet it*
> *tastes like heaven. I tried it for the first time almost*
> *a year ago, because I happened to have all the ingre-*
> *dients in the house. I didn't have particularly high*
> *expectations, but I was completely blown away by it*
> *– as is everyone else I make it for. We now have it at*
> *least once a week – it's become a·staple in our house-*
> *hold. It's probably the best chicken soup I've ever*
> *tasted.*

SERVES FOUR

1 litre chicken stock (or enough to make sure the chicken breasts are covered)

2 chicken breasts

Juice and zest of 1 lemon, cut into thin strips, plus extra juice if needed

Good handful of fresh mint, chopped

100g arborio rice

1. Heat the chicken stock in a large pan and add the chicken breasts, lemon zest and mint. Poach for 10 to 15 minutes, or until chicken is cooked through. Remove the chicken from pan and cut into thin strips.
2. Return the chicken to the pan. Add the rice and lemon juice. Simmer for 20 minutes until the rice is cooked.

Check the seasoning, adding more lemon juice if necessary. Serve immediately.

Nutrition per portion: 179 kcal, protein 19g, carbohydrate 21g, fat 2g, saturated fat 0.3g, fibre 0.5g, sugar 0.3g, salt 2.02g

TUSCAN BEAN SOUP

The Italians know a thing or two about soup and this combination of tomatoes, beans and greens is packed with satisfaction and an abundance of nutrition.

SERVES FOUR
Olive oil
2 rashers of streaky bacon, chopped (optional)
1 onion, finely chopped
2 sticks of celery, diced
1 carrot, diced
2 cloves of garlic, finely sliced
Sprig of rosemary, finely chopped (or a pinch of dried)
300g greens (kale, Swiss chard, spring greens), torn
400g tin of chopped tomatoes
400g tin of beans, drained (cannellini, haricot or flageolet)
1.5 litres vegetable stock
Grated Parmesan (optional)

1. Heat the oil in a heavy-based saucepan, add the bacon, onion, celery, carrot, garlic and rosemary. Cook over a low heat until the onions are a little soft and add the greens.
2. Continue to cook over a low-medium heat until the greens are wilted.
3. Add the tomatoes, a pinch of salt and black pepper and turn up the heat a touch. About 5 minutes later, add the beans and stock, then bring to the boil.
4. Lower the heat, partially cover and simmer for about 30 minutes. You may need to add water if it becomes too thick.

5. Serve sprinkled with Parmesan.

Nutrition per portion: 198 kcal, protein 10g, carbohydrate 26g, fat 7g, saturated fat 0.6g, fibre 8.9g, sugar 11.3g, salt 4.35g

✓ WILD GARLIC SOUP

Every month Luzia Barclay sends out a lovely newsletter on a particular wild herb or food (see Resources). My favourite was when she chose wild garlic:

If you drive or walk through any bit of British woodland in the spring, the chances are that you will notice strong garlic scents on the wind. It seems strange to smell garlic miles away from a kitchen. Wild garlic can be used in salads, soups or mixed with vegetables. It is free food and medicine.

Wild garlic, with its many sulphur compounds, clears the inside of the digestive tract. It detoxifies the gut from pathogens and at the same time supports the 'good' bacteria. It kills many parasites and assists in clearing Candida albicans, a common yeast infection. Wild garlic is a truly versatile plant.

SERVES FOUR
1 tablespoon oil
1 large onion, finely sliced
300g wild garlic
1 litre chicken or vegetable stock
3 tablespoons half-fat crème fraîche

1. Heat up the oil. Fry the onion for a few minutes in the oil until tender, but not brown. Add in the wild garlic and cook for 5 minutes.
2. Pour in the stock and cook on a slow heat for 20 minutes.

3. Blend, add the crème fraîche and adjust the seasoning to your taste. Serve immediately.

Nutrition per portion: 154 kcal, protein 7g, carbohydrate 18g, fat 6g, saturated fat 1.5g, fibre 3.9g, sugar 4.5g, salt 1.93g

Flat Tummy Club Member Soups

Sam's Vietnamese Pho

My Pho recipe is by no means traditional, it's an angli-cized version of the most delicious noodle soup I have ever eaten – usually for breakfast in Hanoi. This soup can be made with beef or shellfish, but chicken is my favourite.

Basically, I make some good chicken stock, shred cooked chicken into it and then add heaps of fresh coriander, chilli, salt, lime, bean sprouts and rice noodles and that is it! This soup is wonderful because you can add to your taste and it really is fabulous to eat and very comforting, at any time of day. It is also light and that's always good.

Katy's chicken soup

I had delicious home-made soup this evening (chicken pieces, chicken stock [home-made], roasted sweetcorn, pearl barley, carrots). How wholesome is that?

✔ Jacq's quick bean soup

Borlotti beans (a tin), garlic, parsley, chicken stock, with some of the beans crushed to make it more solid in the soupy bit, Parmesan. Done.

Sara at the wonderful Goldhill Organic Farm Shop

At lunchtime Michael and I had a head-to-head with squash soup. Mine was squash, cumin, nutmeg and lemon with fresh coriander on top, his was sweet chilli and roasted walnuts. I have never had roasted walnuts before as I am not a walnut fan, but these were great, although we decided my soup was the most warming one. And so this time I won.

CHILLED APPLE SOUP

I went to visit a friend and she promised to make me this soup. It was October when the apples were in peak season. I was a little apprehensive as I'm not a chilled soup fan, but I was won over by its simplicity and subtlety. It's full of Flat Tummy spices in the curry powder and the sprinkle of cayenne and there's lemon juice to boost our digestion and be the perfect partner to the apples.

SERVES FOUR TO SIX
1 onion, sliced
Olive oil
1kg apples (whatever is in season – give them a go!), cored, peeled and quartered
1 heaped teaspoon curry powder
1 litre light chicken or vegetable stock
Juice of ½ a large lemon or 1 small
100ml half-fat crème fraîche
Pinch of cayenne pepper

1. Soften the onion in the olive oil in a big pan for 10 minutes or so while you prepare the apples. After a few minutes, add the curry powder.
2. Add the stock and the apples. Bring up to the boil and then reduce to a simmer for about 30 minutes or until the apples are very soft.
3. Check the seasoning, purée in a blender and pass this through a sieve.
4. Once the soup has cooled, add the lemon juice and crème fraîche. Check the seasoning and serve at room

temperature (or chilled if you prefer) with a tiny dusting of cayenne pepper.

Nutrition per portion: 202 kcal, protein 3g, carbohydrate 33g, fat 8g, saturated fat 2.8g, fibre 4.9g, sugar 30.6g, salt 1.02g

WARM CURRIED CELERIAC SOUP

This soup came about after a visit to a farm shop one October weekend. Celeriac is a weird-looking, gnarled root vegetable, which has a lovely subtle taste that combines celery and parsley. It's a fantastic alternative to white potatoes, making a delicious mash.

SERVES THREE

Olive oil

1 onion, sliced

½ teaspoon ground turmeric

½ teaspoon curry powder

Sea salt and freshly ground black pepper

600g peeled celeriac, chopped into large chunks

1 sweet cooking apple, cored, peeled and roughly chopped

600ml light chicken or vegetable stock

1 tablespoon lemon juice

1. Gently soften the onion in the olive oil in a big saucepan and add the spices and black pepper.
2. After a few minutes, add the celeriac, cover the pan and leave for a few minutes.
3. Add the apple and the stock, bring to the boil and then reduce to a simmer for about 20 minutes or until the apple and celeriac are soft.
4. Add the lemon juice, purée the soup in a blender and check seasoning before serving.

Nutrition per portion: 117 kcal, protein 3g, carbohydrate 15g, fat 5g, saturated fat 0.5g, fibre 9g, sugar 11.7g, salt 1.24g

ROASTED TOMATO AND BASIL SOUP

Tomatoes, olive oil and herbs – the perfect Mediterranean combination and full of ingredients for a Flat Tummy, from the lemon zest to the leek.

SERVES THREE

500g ripe vine tomatoes, quartered (or whole cherry tomatoes)
2 tablespoons extra-virgin olive oil
1 tablespoon chopped thyme
2 teaspoons grated lemon zest
1 leek, chopped
2 cloves of garlic, chopped
1 small glass of white wine (optional)
500ml vegetable stock
1 tablespoon lemon juice (about ½ lemon)
2 tablespoons torn basil

1. Preheat the oven to 230°C/450°F/gas 8.
2. Place the tomatoes in one layer on a baking sheet. Drizzle about 1 tablespoon olive oil onto the tomatoes and sprinkle over the thyme, lemon zest and a little sea salt. Roast for about 30 minutes until the tomatoes are charred and very soft.
3. In a big saucepan, fry the leek and garlic for a few minutes in the rest of the olive oil. Add the wine and boil for a couple of minutes, then add the tomatoes and stock. Bring to the boil, cover and simmer for 10 minutes.
4. Add the lemon juice and purée in a blender. Check for seasoning and serve with the torn basil stirred through.

Nutrition per portion: 119 kcal, protein 2g, carbohydrate 8g, fat 9g, saturated fat 1.1g, fibre 2.8g, sugar 6.3g, salt 1.74g

HOT CUCUMBER SOUP

Cucumber is not the most exciting vegetable, but it's a natural diuretic and so helps with water retention. It also works surprisingly well in this punchy soup, a good balance for all the strong flavours.

SERVES TWO

500ml light chicken stock
80g Italian farro (or pearl barley)
1 lemongrass stalk, bashed
4-6 spring onions, chopped
1 medium cucumber, peeled, deseeded and sliced into rough chunks on the diagonal
1 red chilli (or to taste), deseeded and finely sliced
Soy sauce, to taste
Freshly ground black pepper
2 tablespoons half-fat crème fraîche
1 thumb of fresh ginger, peeled and thinly sliced

1. Bring the stock to the boil and add the farro and lemongrass. Lower to a simmer until the grains are cooked (see the packet instructions), but still with a little bite.
2. Add the spring onion, cucumber and chilli. Simmer for a couple of minutes, and then add the soy sauce and black pepper, to taste.
3. Bring off the heat, leave for a couple of minutes, and then stir through the crème fraîche. Serve with a generous sprinkle of fresh ginger, removing the lemongrass.

Nutrition per portion: 199 kcal, protein 5g, carbohydrate 38g, fat 4g, saturated fat 1.6g, fibre 1.1g, sugar 3g, salt 1.12g

Salads

We've come a long way from lettuce, cucumber and tomato . . . although a simple tomato and onion salad with balsamic and extra-virgin olive oil while on holiday in southern Italy can't really be surpassed!

It's the little extras that can make a salad, from a sprinkle of toasted pine nuts to a tangy lemon dressing. A friend of mine serves a big green salad with dinner every night and it's the perfect way to fit another portion of leaves into your day. Or you might fancy starting your supper with a simple rocket salad, although I'm a bit spoilt now that I've eaten rocket from the farm near my parents. They allow the rocket to get much bigger than we are used to seeing in the supermarkets and so it has a lovely mild taste and doesn't get stuck in your teeth.

Packed Lunch Combos

1 medium avocado, 50g smoked salmon and salad leaves with a squeeze of lemon juice and freshly ground black pepper

Salade Niçoise – ½ can of tuna steak in spring water, green leaves, tomatoes, green beans and a hard-boiled egg

Wild rice (about 40g dry weight, follow the cooking instructions on the packet), beetroot and smoked trout (½ a pack, approximately 60g)

Poached salmon (about 100g) and watercress with lots of lemon juice and black pepper

Chicken (about 150g) with leftover roasted vegetables and quinoa (about 40g dry weight, follow the cooking instructions on the packet)

½ pack (100g) frozen cooked and peeled large king prawns (defrosted), medium avocado, a little mayonnaise (about a teaspoon), lemon juice, favourite salad leaves and lots of torn basil

✓ SUPERFOOD SALAD (INSPIRED BY LEON)

I love Leon – a healthy fast food restaurant chain that has made quinoa and brown rice trendy and tasty. This is an homage to their classic Superfood Salad, which is a combination of so many Flat Tummy foods. Even the cheese is goat's cheese, thought to be more easily digested than cow's. It has such a lovely strong taste you only need a little.

SERVES ONE

Cucumber sticks (if cucumber gives you indigestion, try peeling it and see if that helps)

Medium avocado, sliced

40g quinoa (dry weight), cooked (follow the cooking instructions on the packet)

25g goat's cheese, crumbled

1 tablespoon mixed seeds

FOR THE DRESSING

1 tablespoon olive oil

Lemon juice, to taste

Freshly ground black pepper

Mix it all together!

Nutrition per portion: 612 kcal, protein 14g, carbohydrate 29g, fat 50g, saturated fat 8g, fibre 6g, sugar 5g, salt 0.34g

✓ POACHED CHICKEN AND MINT SALAD

This salad from Dawn combines lean protein with lots of vegetables, seeds for added essential fats and zingy fresh Asian flavours.

SERVES TWO
500ml water or chicken stock
2 skinless chicken breasts
¼ cabbage, finely shredded
1 carrot, cut into matchsticks
4 spring onions, sliced into strips
1 small handful of mint, roughly chopped
1 teaspoon sesame seeds
Soy sauce

FOR THE DRESSING
2 tablespoons lime juice
1 teaspoon agave syrup or honey
1 tablespoon fish sauce

1. Bring the water or stock to the boil and then poach the chicken breasts for 10 to 15 minutes at a simmer, until the chicken is cooked through. Remove the chicken from the water/stock and leave to cool.
2. Shred the chicken and add to the veg and mint.
3. Mix the dressing, pour over the salad, toss and scatter over the sesame seeds.
4. Drizzle soy sauce over the top when all assembled.

Nutrition per portion: 221 kcal, protein 38g, carbohydrate 11g, fat 3g, saturated fat 0.7g, fibre 3.8g, sugar 10g, salt 2.12g

SALMON AND PRAWN MOUSSE

This recipe from Caroline is the perfect summer Sunday lunch alternative.

SERVES FOUR
500g salmon
A few sprigs of dill
2 lemons
1 packet (7g) of powdered gelatine
2 tablespoons mayonnaise (low-fat if preferred)
2 tablespoons half-fat crème fraîche
Sea salt and white pepper
Squeeze of tomato ketchup
Tabasco
1 teaspoon horseradish sauce
150g cooked and peeled king prawns

1. Preheat the oven to 180°C/350°F/gas 4.
2. Place the salmon in lightly oiled foil with the sprigs of dill and slices of one of the lemons. Make a parcel, place on a baking tray and cook in the oven for 20 minutes.
3. Meanwhile, dissolve the gelatine in about 100ml of water, just off the boil. Set aside to cool while the fish cooks.
4. When the fish is cooked, place in a bowl and flake it quite finely, but do not mash it.
5. Mix together the mayonnaise, crème fraîche, salt, white pepper, juice of the remaining lemon, ketchup, a shake of Tabasco, the horseradish sauce and the cooled gelatin. Stir in the flaked salmon and the prawns. Scoop all into a bowl and place in the fridge to set.

6. When set, turn the bowl upside down and gently shake out the mousse to serve.

7. Decorate the mousse with peeled, deseeded and chopped cucumber tossed with a little olive oil and dill and you have an excellent lunch dish that you can serve with a Summer Salad (see page 296).

Nutrition per portion: 308 kcal, protein 36g, carbohydrate 2g, fat 17g, saturated fat 3.9g, fibre 0.1g, sugar 1.7g, salt 1.66g

✓ SUMMER SALAD

Here is a lovely way to combine any combination of peas, broad beans, mangetout, sugar snaps, fine green beans or asparagus with salad leaves for a bowl of delicious healthiness. Caroline, who sent in this simple but gorgeous recipe, suggests you choose three veggies from the list in equal quantity, about 50g of each vegetable per person. The peas and broad beans can be frozen, but fresh are tastier.

SERVES THREE

450g peas, broad beans, mangetout, sugar snaps, fine
    green beans or asparagus
1 lemon
2 cloves of garlic
Extra-virgin olive oil
Handful of mint, chopped
Sea salt and freshly ground black pepper
1 bag (80-100g) green salad leaves
Balsamic vinegar (it is worth buying good balsamic vine-
    gar for its depth of flavour and lack of sharpness)

Cooking times for vegetables vary a little according to how old the vegetables are. Check ahead of time so you don't overcook them. Ideally, they will be tender, but still crisp with a little bite.

Peas – 3 to 5 minutes
Broad beans (podded) – 1 to 3 minutes
Mangetout – 2 to 3 minutes
Sugar snap peas – 3 to 4 minutes
Green beans – 5 minutes
Asparagus – 4 to 8 minutes

1. If using asparagus or beans, chop them into two or three pieces. Cook your vegetables separately until just cooked, drain and quickly refresh in cold water to stop them cooking and to maintain their green colour. If the broad beans are rather large, slip them out of their skins and just use the soft inner part.

2. Using a sharp knife or potato peeler, pare some strips of peel from the lemon and chop the garlic cloves into two or three pieces each. Toss your cooked vegetables in the olive oil – the quantity depends on the volume of vegetables, but you want them lightly coated all over. Now mix in the garlic, lemon peel and some freshly chopped mint. Season lightly. This can all be covered with clingfilm and placed in the fridge until needed – overnight is fine.

3. Shortly before serving, place your green salad leaves in a bowl. Take the lemon peel and garlic pieces out of the vegetable mix and discard. Put the vegetables with the leaves and drizzle a little balsamic vinegar over the salad.

Nutrition per portion: 162 kcal, protein 9g, carbohydrate 13g, fat 9g, saturated fat 1.4g, fibre 6.8g, sugar 4.5g, salt 0.51g

✓ SPICY BEEF SALAD

I don't eat masses of red meat, but a little quality beef from grass-fed cattle is a good source of protein and spicing it up in a salad is a great alternative to chips!

SERVES TWO
2 lime leaves, finely chopped or the grated zest of 1 lime
1 handful of mint leaves, chopped
1 handful of coriander leaves, chopped
¼ cucumber, peeled and cut into matchsticks
1 carrot, peeled and cut into matchsticks
8 cherry tomatoes
Bunch of watercress
2 small sirloin or rump steaks
1 tablespoon olive oil
Sea salt and freshly ground black pepper

FOR THE DRESSING
1 small, very hot chilli, deseeded and very finely chopped
Juice of 1 lime
Pinch of sugar
2 tablespoons Thai fish sauce
1½ teaspoons sweet chilli sauce

1. First, make the dressing. Mix the chilli in a bowl with the lime juice, sugar, fish sauce and chilli sauce.
2. Put the lime leaves or grated zest into a bowl, then add the mint and coriander. Add the cucumber and carrot matchsticks to the herb mix. Halve the tomatoes, pick over the watercress, wash it and add both to the bowl. Now toss the salad with the dressing and divide between two plates.

3. Rub the steaks with a little oil, season lightly, then grill or griddle them to taste – only a few minutes each side for rare, a little more for better done. Leave to rest for a couple of minutes, then slice them into thick strips and lay these over the salad on each plate.

Nutrition per portion: 353 kcal, protein 36g, carbohydrate 10g, fat 19g, saturated fat 7.3g, fibre 2.3g, sugar 8.3g, salt 3.9g

TOMATO AND CUCUMBER SALAD

This is so simple, but delicious and fresh. It does require salt to remove some of the moisture of the cucumber, so save this recipe for a hot summer's day when your body needs it. This is the perfect accompaniment to cold chicken or poached salmon. Simply make as much as you fancy.

Cucumber
Sea salt and freshly ground black pepper
Tomatoes
Lemon juice
Chives, finely chopped

1. Peel and finely slice the cucumber. Place in a colander and sprinkle with salt. Set aside for 30 minutes, then rinse under the tap and blot thoroughly dry with kitchen roll.
2. With a knife, take out the green eye of the tomatoes if they look coarse and place in a bowl. Pour over boiling water and leave for 30 seconds. Run under cold water, peel away the skins and finely slice.
3. Using an open dish, layer the vegetables alternately. Season vigorously with black pepper, but not salt as the cucumber will have a residual saltiness. Squeeze over the juice of a lemon and finish by sprinkling with the chives.

Nutrition per portion: 42 kcal, protein 2g, carbohydrate 7g, fat 1g, saturated fat 0.1g, fibre 2.4g, sugar 6.9g, salt 0.8g

TOMATOES

I have a friend who, like me, is a real fusspot about tomatoes. We have a laugh describing how we'd always have to pull the tomato out of sandwiches as kids and still do, and have to buy the most expensive tinned tomatoes as there is always less skin to pick out. But I do love good tomatoes and they are super healthy too. The deeper the colour, the more lycopene they contain, which has been shown to have antioxidant, cancer-preventing and heart disease-preventing properties. Originally tomatoes came from South America, but of course now they make us think of sunny days in the Mediterranean. I always have a spicy tomato juice on the plane; it's funny how so many people do, and yet I don't think to make it at home. It would be the perfect Flat Tummy snack!

✓ HUMMUS

Caroline told me her recipe for hummus is better than shop-bought and I have to agree. The chickpeas are a great source of protein and fibre, while the tahini, made from sesame seeds, is rich in minerals like magnesium and calcium. This is perfect for lunch with the Grated Carrot Salad (see page 295) or vegetable crudités and a slice of soda bread.

SERVES FOUR
400g tin of chickpeas
4 tablespoons olive oil
4 tablespoons tahini (about 40g)
3-4 tablespoons lemon juice
2 cloves of garlic
Sea salt and freshly ground black pepper

1. Drain the chickpeas, but reserve the liquid.
2. Place the chickpeas, oil, tahini, 3 spoons of the lemon juice and the garlic into a food processor and whizz until smooth, adding the chickpea liquid as needed to acquire the right consistency.
3. Taste, season and add more lemon juice if needed.
4. Serve with the carrot salad.

Nutrition per portion: 232 kcal, protein 6g, carbohydrate 10g, fat 19g, saturated fat 2.4g, fibre 3.4g, sugar 0.5g, salt 0.84g

✔ GRATED CARROT SALAD

The humble carrot, great value for money and yes, they really do help you see in the dark.

SERVES THREE AS A SIDE
3 carrots
1 shallot, very finely chopped
Drizzle (1 tablespoon) of sunflower or olive oil
Lemon juice, to taste
Pinch of sea salt and a pinch of sugar (depending on your
    carrots)

1. Preferably using a food processor, grate the carrots as finely as possible.
2. Now mix with the other ingredients. If your carrots are young, they will not need the sugar as they will be sweet enough; if they are older, they may need a pinch. Leave to soften a while before serving.

Nutrition per portion: 65 kcal, protein 1g, carbohydrate 7g, fat 4g, saturated fat 0.5g, fibre 2.1g, sugar 6.9g, salt 0.14g

✓ CUMIN LENTIL SALAD

Lentils have a nutty flavour and are a rich source of protein, a great alternative to meat. I can find them overpowering on the plate, but thanks to my dad and FTC member Caroline, I have been won over and now have a recipe that strikes the perfect balance between the flavours of the dressing and the lentils.

SERVES FOUR
240g green or Puy lentils
Pinch of sea salt
4 tablespoons olive oil
Juice of ½ to 1 lemon
Pepper
1 teaspoon ground cumin
5 spring onions, finely chopped
Small bunch of parsley or mint

1. Simmer the lentils in enough water to cover them for 20 to 30 minutes until tender, adding a little salt towards the end.
2. Drain and mix with the remaining ingredients straight-away so the hot lentils absorb the dressing.
3. Serve warm or cold.

Nutrition per portion: 284 kcal, protein 15g, carbohydrate 30g, fat 12g, saturated fat 1.5g, fibre 5.6g, sugar 1.1g, salt 0.11g

✓ BEETROOT AND FETA COUSCOUS

This recipe was adapted from one of those very handy supermarket recipe cards, in this instance Waitrose. Like the Sunday supplements, they are a great source of ideas.

SERVES TWO

4 medium or 2 large beetroots, peeled and chopped for roasting

1 tablespoon olive oil

Sea salt and freshly ground black pepper

80g couscous (dry weight), cooked (follow the cooking instructions on the packet)

60g feta, crumbled

Sprinkling of toasted almond flakes

Handful of mint, torn

FOR THE DRESSING

2 tablespoons olive oil

1 teaspoon ground cinnamon

Juice and zest of 1 orange

1. Drizzle a little olive oil over the beetroot in a roasting tray, season, cover with foil and bake at 180°C/350°F/gas 4 for 30 to 45 minutes or until you can easily pierce with a fork.
2. Prepare your couscous according to the packet and share between the plates.
3. Mix all the dressing ingredients together.
4. When the beetroot is cooked, simply add to the couscous along with the feta, almond flakes, mint and dressing.

Nutrition per portion: 431 kcal, protein 12g, carbohydrate 41g, fat 26g, saturated fat 6.4g, fibre 4.1g, sugar 18g, salt 1.64g

Dressings

With around 120 calories in a tablespoon of vegetable or nut oil, it's a good Flat Tummy idea to check how much dressing you tend to add to a salad or recipe. You might even use a tablespoon rather than pour direct from the bottle or jug, just while you are getting used to the idea of what's a healthy amount. When making dressings, always think about how you can add other ingredients to bulk out any oil. Here are just a few ideas to get your creative juices flowing:

Extra-virgin olive oil, lemon juice, thyme, sea salt and freshly ground black pepper, to taste

Extra-virgin olive oil, lemon balm, red wine vinegar, sea salt and freshly ground black pepper, to taste

Sesame oil, lime juice, tamari (a Japanese soy sauce), sea salt and freshly ground black pepper, to taste

Extra-virgin olive oil, lemon or orange juice, agave syrup or honey and freshly ground black pepper

Avocado oil, lemon juice, sea salt and freshly ground black pepper

Apple cider vinegar, honey and mustard, sea salt and freshly ground black pepper, to taste

Raspberry vinegar, extra-virgin olive oil, Dijon mustard, sea salt and freshly ground black pepper, to taste

Umeboshi vinegar, sesame oil, lemon juice, sea salt and freshly ground black pepper, to taste

Main Meals

Enjoy a balance of light, fresh suppers with hearty meals thrown in on occasion. Go for lean proteins, lots of whole grains and whatever vegetables are in season. A friend of my mum's was on a diet where she couldn't eat anything orange, how bizarre is that? I say enjoy as much variety as possible.

For those evenings when you get home exhausted or too late to cook, here are a few ideas to steer you away from the takeaway menus and ready meals.

Ultra Easy 'Assembly' Meals

Always have a pot of soup in the fridge, home-made or from the chilled aisle

Chilled cooked trout, mackerel or salmon with salad

Couscous takes literally 5 minutes and zero effort. With a squeeze of lemon juice and whatever herbs you have to hand, it's a healthy side dish for leftover chicken, a quick grilled fillet of salmon or a couple of slices of proper ham and salad

Scrambled eggs on wholegrain toast with tomatoes

Freeze individual portions of stews and always have a few fresh or frozen vegetables as stand-bys. You'll have a home-cooked meal ready with no effort in less than 10 minutes

Stir-fry some prawns or chicken with ready-prepared vegetables, a splash of soy sauce and a squeeze of lemon or lime

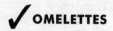 OMELETTES

Eggs are satisfying and a great source of protein. My mum makes a lovely omelette and her two top tips are don't over-whisk the eggs or you can end up with a rubbery omelette and wait until the pan (which should be small) is really hot.

SERVES ONE
2 large organic eggs
Freshly ground black pepper
½ teaspoon butter or 1 teaspoon olive oil

DELICIOUS FILLING COMBINATIONS
Goat's cheese and thyme
Smoked salmon and a little cream cheese
Ham and mushrooms (I cook the mushrooms first in the same pan) with some chopped herbs if I have anything fresh to hand
Plain with a cherry tomato and basil salad

1. Whisk the eggs and add plenty of freshly ground black pepper.
2. Melt the butter or heat the oil in a non-stick frying pan. Pour in the eggs and cook quickly on a high heat, letting any uncooked egg run over the edges of the cooked egg. I like a soft omelette, so add the other ingredients after about 2 minutes and before the egg is completely set. Fold over the omelette in the pan before sliding out onto a waiting warm plate.

Nutrition per portion (plain omlette only): 200 kcal, protein 15g, carbohydrate 0g, fat 16g, saturated fat 4.9g, fibre 0g, sugar 0g, salt 0.47g

✓ ASPARAGUS WITH AN EGG

1. Steam a big bunch of asparagus (with the woody ends snapped off) for about 5 minutes until tender, poach an egg and pop it on top. If you aren't confident poaching eggs, then fry an egg in a little olive oil. Poaching is more healthy as you don't add any oil; the easiest way to poach an egg is as follows:
2. Use a very fresh egg and crack into a tea cup.
3. Bring a saucepan of water to the boil, but then reduce to a low simmer so that you can see the bubbles on the bottom and there is just a hint of movement in the water.
4. Gently slide the egg into the water and poach for 3 minutes if using a medium egg. Keep an eye on the water to make sure it doesn't start to boil.
5. Remove the water from the heat and use a slotted spoon to remove the egg. Pop the egg on some kitchen towel, just to soak up the excess water, and serve.

Nutrition per portion: 129 kcal, protein 15g, carbohydrate 5g, fat 7g, saturated fat 1.5g, fibre 3.8g, sugar 4.3g, salt 0.18g

✓ ASPARAGUS WITH FETA AND PEAS

SERVES ONE
100g asparagus, with the woody ends snapped off
100g frozen peas
1 tablespoon olive oil
1 teaspoon lemon juice
Freshly ground black pepper
50g feta cheese, crumbled
A few fresh mint leaves, torn (optional)

1. Steam the asparagus for about 5 minutes until tender and boil the frozen peas for a couple of minutes.
2. Mix the olive oil and lemon juice together with some freshly ground black pepper.
3. Toss the asparagus, peas, crumbled feta and dressing together and sprinkle over a few torn mint leaves if using.

Nutrition per portion: 316 kcal, protein 16g, carbohydrate 12g, fat 23g, saturated fat 8.2g, fibre 6.8g, sugar 5.3g, salt 1.34g

ASPARAGUS

Early British asparagus hits the shops around May. Delicious and versatile, asparagus packs quite a nutritious punch. According to British Asparagus, it is one of the richest sources of rutin, which together with vitamin C can help to energize and protect the body from infections. It is a source of iron and low in calories, with an average of less than 4 calories per spear. Low in cholesterol, fat-free and a mild diuretic, asparagus is believed to help detoxify the body and get rid of excess water. Asparagus also contains prebiotics, good for the tummy and digestion. I have simple tastes and love steamed asparagus with a poached egg on top. Here are a few more ideas from my Flat Tummy friend and foodie Camilla:

I like eating asparagus with balsamic vinegar, a little olive oil, shaves of Parmesan (a bit of strong cheese goes a long way as we know) and lots of salt and pepper. I also like a poached egg on top of a steamed bundle or to use them as soldiers, dipped into a soft-boiled egg. I like chopped asparagus added to a big green salad with crisp-fried Parma ham broken into shards and any other brightly coloured, crunchy salad things I might have in my fridge. Sometimes I steam some asparagus and, when cold, roll each one in a piece of Parma ham. These then go in my trusty Tupperware for my packed lunch. So nothing very original, but all pleasurable, especially if you use your fingers, which I always think makes food taste better.

✓ LEMON AND GINGER SALMON

Salmon gets its fair share of good and bad press in terms of how it is farmed and, as a consequence, whether it's good for us to eat. As with everything, perhaps if we enjoy a variety of fresh fish, asking the fishmonger what's looking particularly good on the day and what they'd recommend, we'll strike a healthy balance. Like all oily fish, salmon is packed with essential fats and is so versatile when it comes to cooking. I often have this with some bulgur wheat, steamed pak choy and a little soy sauce drizzled over everything (and another squeeze of lemon juice). Quick, easy and delicious!

SERVES ONE
1 small/medium salmon fillet
½ teaspoon of grated fresh ginger
Juice and grated zest of ½ lemon
Sea salt and freshly ground black pepper

1. Cover the top of the salmon fillet with the ginger, lemon zest and juice and season.
2. Place on foil and grill for approximately 8 to 10 minutes skin side down, and then skin side up for just a couple of minutes.

Nutrition per portion: 254 kcal, protein 28g, carbohydrate 0g, fat 15g, saturated fat 3.1g, fibre 0g, sugar 0.1g, salt 0.66g

✓ SEA BASS AND LEMONY LEEKS

Unlike French women, I don't eat leek soup to get a flatter tummy, but I am happy to eat a mound of them, in this case beneath a lovely piece of bass.

PER PERSON
A little butter (about 15g)
1 leek, sliced
1 good-sized sea bass fillet
Sea salt and freshly ground black pepper
Fine oatmeal or flour, for dusting
1 tablespoon olive oil
Lemon juice
2 tablespoons half-fat crème fraîche

1. Melt the butter in a non-stick saucepan and add the leek, gently softening over a low heat for about 10 minutes.
2. Season and dust the sea bass with a little flour (I like to use fine oatmeal, but not essential). Heat the olive oil in a non-stick frying pan and cook the sea bass, skin side first, for about 5 minutes. Add a good squeeze of lemon, turn the fillet over and then take off the heat.
3. Stir the crème fraîche into the leeks and add plenty of freshly ground black pepper and another squeeze of lemon. Serve the sea bass on top of a bed of leeks.

Nutrition per portion: 677 kcal, protein 72g, carbohydrate 13g, fat 38g, saturated fat 13.9g, fibre 3.4g, sugar 4g, salt 1.43g

✓ JERK TUNA

Among other things, jerk seasoning contains cinnamon and chilli, both excellent Flat Tummy spices. And tuna is a fantastic oily fish to cook on the rare side, just be sure that the fishmonger can recommend a really fresh piece for you.

SERVES TWO
2 tuna steaks
Jerk seasoning (available in supermarkets)
Lemon

1. Coat the tuna steaks in the jerk seasoning and, if time allows, set aside for a while.
2. Place the steaks under a hot grill. Cook for a couple of minutes each side, depending on the thickness, as tuna is best kept a little pink in the middle.
3. Serve with lemon and a green salad.

Nutrition per portion: 200 kcal, protein 33g, carbohydrate 2g, fat 7g, saturated fat 1.5g, fibre 0g, sugar 0.8g, salt 0.24g

JO AND DAWN'S MISO SALMON

The marinade is a Jo Pratt creation and the rice combination is what my friend Dawn had to hand – the perfect mix.

SERVES ONE
1 teaspoon miso paste
1 teaspoon honey
1 teaspoon mirin
1 medium salmon fillet
40g jasmine rice
A few leaves of fresh mint and coriander, chopped
Soy sauce, to taste
2–3 spring onions, chopped

1. Mix up the first three ingredients in a bowl and smear over the salmon fillet. Let the salmon marinate for half an hour.
2. Cook the rice according to the packet instructions while the salmon is marinating.
3. Pop the salmon on a baking tray and grill under a high heat for 5 to 6 minutes (or until the salmon is cooked).
4. Stir the herbs through the rice and serve the salmon on top, drizzled with soy sauce and scattered with the chopped spring onions.

Nutrition per portion: 423 kcal, protein 32g, carbohydrate 40g, fat 16g, saturated fat 3.1g, fibre 0.4g, sugar 4.9g, salt 0.95g

✓ GINGER AND SESAME PRAWN STIR-FRY

This is one of those store cupboard recipes that only takes a few minutes to pull together, but is a burst of flavours. Use any veg you have to hand that can take a bit of vigorous stir-frying. I always keep jumbo prawns in the freezer as a stand-by, especially as they always seem to be on special offer. Prawns are a great source of protein for hardly any fat or calories.

SERVES ONE
½ pack (100g) frozen large raw king prawns (defrosted)
1 or 2 pak choy, roughly chopped
½ courgette, chopped
FOR THE MARINADE
Fresh ginger, crushed or finely sliced, to taste (I have about 1 teaspoon)
Clove of garlic, crushed
Zest and juice of ½ lemon
1½ tablespoons soy sauce
½ tablespoon mirin
1 tablespoon agave syrup or honey
½ tablespoon sesame oil (if you're not keen, any type of nut oil)

1. Combine all the ingredients for the marinade in a large bowl.
2. Add the prawns and veg to the bowl and mix thoroughly.
3. Heat a wok to a high heat and simply add the mixed prawns and vegetables and stir-fry for 5 minutes. This dish doesn't need any noodles or rice with it.

Nutrition per portion: 249 kcal, protein 26g, carbohydrate 22g, fat 7g, saturated fat 1g, fibre 1.6g, sugar 16.5g, salt 6g

STIR-FRY COMBINATIONS

My sister has two teenage, very sporty sons who never stop eating. Stir-fries have become a firm favourite with the whole family as my sister can give them extra big portions of noodles or rice while she tends to have more veggies.

Mix and match your own combination

Protein	Vegetables	Flavours
Tofu	Tenderstem broccoli	Ginger
Chicken	Purple sprouting broccoli	Lemon
Turkey	Mushrooms	Lime
Pork	Spring onions	Chilli
Prawns	Pak choy	Soy sauce
Tuna	Cabbage	Mirin
Salmon	Bean sprouts	Fish sauce
	Carrot	Sesame oil
	Courgette	Honey
		Green curry paste
		Coconut milk

✓ MEDITERRANEAN ROASTED FISH

This is a very pretty dish that combines a lovely white fish with olive oil, lemon and herbs, all good for a Flat Tummy.

SERVES TWO
2 whole bream, sea bass or mullet
2 tablespoons olive oil
1 lemon
6 bay leaves
Several pinches of dried oregano
Sea salt and freshly ground black pepper

1. Set the oven at 240°C/475°F/gas 9.
2. Rinse and pat dry the fish using kitchen roll, then lay it flat in a baking dish. (Useful tip – if you line the dish with greaseproof paper, the fish will not stick to the bottom).
3. Shake a little olive oil over the fish and squeeze over the lemon juice. Chop up the remains of the lemon and lay the pieces around the fish with the bay leaves and oregano, then season with sea salt and black pepper.
4. Timing depends on the size of your fish, but place in the oven for 20 minutes and then test to see if the flesh comes away from the bone easily – if not, put it back for a few more minutes.
5. Serve with more lemon and steamed veggies for the perfect Flat Tummy combination.

Nutrition per portion: 393 kcal, protein 53g, carbohydrate 1g, fat 20g, saturated fat 3.2g, fibre 0g, sugar 0.8g, salt 1.34g

MONKFISH STEW WITH WARMING HERBS AND SPICES

Monkfish is a meaty fish that can take some pretty robust flavours alongside it. This slightly spicy stew I made towards the end of summer went down a treat and I simply served it with a big pile of sauted chard, full of rainbow colours and packed with nutrients.

SERVES TWO
1 small onion, chopped
1 teaspoon olive oil
1 clove of garlic, finely chopped
1 leek, roughly chopped
1 courgette, roughly chopped
½ teaspoon ground turmeric
½ teaspoon fresh ginger, finely chopped
½ teaspoon mustard seeds
200g passata
100ml vegetable stock
Bay leaf
Fresh thyme or rosemary, or whatever you have to hand
200g monkfish, chopped into 2.5cm square chunks
100g chard

1. Slowly sweat the onion in the olive oil in a big pan and then add the garlic to soften.
2. Add the leek, courgette, turmeric, ginger and mustard seeds and stir in. Leave to infuse for a couple of minutes.
3. Add the passata and enough vegetable stock to just cover the veg.
4. Add the bay leaf and fresh herbs and simmer gently for about 20 minutes.
5. Add the monkfish for about 6 to 7 minutes at the end. To

test the fish is cooked, cut into a piece – it should be opaque, but still moist inside.

6. In the meantime, chop up the chard, wash and then simply sauté in a non-stick pan. The residual water on the chard from rinsing is enough to cook it.

7. Dish up the stew in shallow bowls with the chard on the side.

Nutrition per portion: 178 kcal, protein 21g, carbohydrate 15g, fat 4g, saturated fat 0.5g, fibre 2.8g, sugar 7.9g, salt 1.34g

TUNA WITH FENNEL-ROASTED BEETROOT

The good thing about roasted vegetables is that you can be adventurous with your marinades, from sweet honey and thyme to this spicy combination of turmeric and fennel seeds.

SERVES TWO
3 tablespoons olive oil
½ tablespoon ground turmeric
¼ teaspoon fennel seeds
2 large carrots, peeled and cut into chunks
1 beetroot, peeled and cut into chunks
Sea salt and freshly ground black pepper
2 medium tuna steaks
Juice of ½ lemon

1. Preheat the oven to 200°C/400°F/gas 6.
2. Mix 2 tablespoons of the olive oil, turmeric and fennel seeds in a large bowl. Add the carrot and beetroot and toss until coated.
3. Place the veg in a shallow baking tray, add 5mm water and sprinkle with sea salt and freshly ground black pepper. Roast for about 45 minutes until the carrots are a little caramelized and the beetroot can be easily pierced with a sharp knife or fork.
4. Season the tuna steaks and rub the remaining olive oil onto each side. Sear the tuna steaks in a non-stick pan over a medium-high heat for just a couple of minutes each side. The thicker the steaks, the longer they will need, but I like tuna to be seared on the outside and pink in the middle.
5. Serve the tuna and veg with the lemon juice drizzled over.

Nutrition per portion: 424 kcal, protein 35g, carbohydrate 18g, fat 24g, saturated fat 3.8g, fibre 4.8g, sugar 15.5g, salt 0.86g

✓ BRAZILIAN PRAWNS

Prawns, lime, ginger, chilli, coriander and coconut . . . a classic South American, and very healthy, combination. Coconut is an interesting food in that the juice is said to be more hydrating than water and the oil in coconut is saturated, yet many nutritionists believe it is good for you and even helps in losing weight. I'm more than happy to test the theory.

If you make this quite soupy, then brown rice works really well. If you are using white basmati, then I think less liquid is best as the rice can go a bit mushy. The quantities are flexible so, for example, I quite often add in more tomato and lots of lime.

SERVES TWO

80g basmati or brown rice
1 pack (200g) raw peeled king prawns
1 lime
Olive oil
2 cloves of garlic, crushed
Knob of fresh ginger (about 2cm squared), grated
1 onion, chopped
½ red pepper, chopped
1 beef tomato, chopped
1 red chilli (seeds in or out, depending on how brave you are!), chopped
Bunch of coriander, finely chopped
50ml coconut cream
50ml fish stock

1. Start cooking the rice according to the packet instructions.
2. Marinate the prawns in the juice of half the lime.

3. Heat the olive oil in a pan – a sauté pan is best – and add in the garlic and ginger, if using. Once the garlic is taking on colour, add in the onion. After a couple of minutes, add the pepper, tomato, chilli and coriander.

4. After about 10 minutes, add the coconut cream and fish stock. Once the liquid has come to the boil and simmered for about 5 minutes, add in the prawns and lime juice and cook until the prawns have turned pink, which should only take about 5 minutes, depending on the size of the prawns. Do not cook for too long otherwise the prawns will go rubbery.

5. Serve on a bed of rice and squeeze some lime juice over just before eating.

Nutrition per portion: 428 kcal, protein 24g, carbohydrate 44g, fat 18g, saturated fat 8.8g, fibre 2.9g, sugar 10g, salt 0.79g

LEMON AND HERB CHICKEN

Thanks again to Caroline Scott-Gall for this reminder of how lemon and herbs make such a good combination. It is so easy, but so tasty. If you are in your weight loss phase, then enjoy this with some lovely purple sprouting broccoli. If you are maintaining your healthy weight, then feel free to add a few new potatoes.

SERVES TWO
4 chicken pieces (thighs work well here)
Finely grated zest and juice of 1 lemon
Handful of mixed, chopped fresh herbs, such as tarragon, parsley, oregano and thyme OR you can use dried herbs in a slightly smaller quantity
Sea salt and freshly ground black pepper

1. Preheat the oven to 200°C/400°F/gas 6.
2. Rub the lemon zest and juice into the chicken with the herbs and add some seasoning.
4. Cook for 30 minutes until crispy on the outside. Serve, not forgetting to scoop up the juices from the pan.

Nutrition per portion: 554 kcal, protein 44g, carbohydrate 1g, fat 41g, saturated fat 12.2g, fibre 0.2g, sugar 0.4g, salt 1.06g

SPICY CHICKEN, FENNEL AND TOMATO

This is a great one-pot meal for during the week and if you have hungry teenagers around, you can always throw a few jacket potatoes in the oven.

SERVES TWO
2 large or 4 small chicken thighs (skinless)
Sea salt and freshly ground black pepper
2 tablespoons groundnut or vegetable oil
Large fennel, sliced
50-75ml vegetable or light chicken stock
400g carton of passata

FOR THE PASTE
2 cardamom pods
½ teaspoon ground cumin
½ teaspoon ground turmeric
¼ teaspoon ground chilli
½ teaspoon mustard (grainy or Dijon, whatever you have)
Drizzle of groundnut oil

1. Season the chicken thighs. Heat the oil in a sauté pan and sauté the chicken until almost browned and cooked through, depending on the size of the thighs, between 10 and 15 minutes.
2. To make the paste, open the cardamom pods and gently release the seeds inside into a pestle and mortar and crush them. Mix in the spices, mustard and groundnut oil, then create a little space on the bottom of the sauté pan and cook the spice paste for a minute or so before mixing into the chicken.
3. Add the sliced fennel and sauté for a couple of minutes

before adding the stock. Simmer for about 5 minutes to begin to soften the fennel.

4. Add the passata (however much you fancy) and bring to a very low simmer for as long as it takes to really soften the fennel and chicken, ideally another 30 minutes.

Nutrition per portion: 413 kcal, protein 44g, carbohydrate 16g, fat 20g, saturated fat 4.5g, fibre 3.5g, sugar 8.6g, salt 2.31g

✓ HARISSA CHICKEN

Harissa paste is a hot combination of tomatoes, very hot chillies and spices like cumin. It's a great store cupboard stand-by for a quick-and-easy dinner.

SERVES TWO
6-8 ripe medium tomatoes, thickly sliced
Sea salt and freshly ground black pepper
Handful of basil, roughly torn
1 tablespoon olive oil
1 tablespoon balsamic vinegar
2 medium skinless and boneless chicken breasts
2 tablespoons natural yoghurt
1 teaspoon harissa paste (available from supermarkets – Belazu make a particularly good one)

1. Preheat the oven to 200°C/400°F/gas 6.
2. Spread the tomatoes in the bottom of an ovenproof dish. Add seasoning, the basil leaves, a little olive oil and balsamic vinegar.
3. Place the chicken on top of the tomatoes. Mix together the yoghurt and harissa paste and spread over the top of the chicken. Now place the dish in the hot oven and cook for 20 minutes. Check to see if the chicken is cooked through by cutting into one of the pieces to ensure there is no pink colour left. If there is, cook for a little longer until done.

Nutrition per portion: 265 kcal, protein 37g, carbohydrate 11g, fat 9g, saturated fat 1.7g, fibre 2.6g, sugar 10.3g, salt 0.85g

ROASTED GUINEA FOWL OR QUAILS

Small birds make for very lean and delicious dinners. And sage is a lovely herb that contains health-giving and brain-boosting antioxidants.

SERVES TWO
1 guinea fowl or 2 quails
A good handful of sage
Sea salt

1. Joint your guinea fowl into four pieces or split your quails by cutting them along the backbone, lying them on a board and pressing down firmly on the breast bone.
2. Spread the sage leaves over the bottom of a roasting tin, put the birds on top, skin side up, and give a good sprinkling of sea salt.
3. Cook for 30 to 40 minutes until crispy on top and falling off the bone. You can test the meat is cooked by piercing with a sharp knife to check the juices run clear.
4. Delicious served with a fruit jelly such as crab apple, roast parsnips and simple seasonal greens.

Nutrition per portion: 237 kcal, protein 25g, carbohydrate 0g, fat 15g, saturated fat 3.8g, fibre 0g, sugar 0g, salt 0.67g

✓ TARRAGON CHICKEN

This is one of my favourite recipes, adapted from *Cook Yourself Thin Quick and Easy* (see Resources). It's extremely easy and quick and the perfect meal for having a quiet night in. You may think the crème fraîche isn't exactly a Flat Tummy ingredient, but half-fat crème fraîche is fantastic for making the occasional dish taste very creamy, while still being good for your waistline.

SERVES TWO
2 medium skinless chicken breasts, chopped into bite-size
Sea salt and freshly ground black pepper
1 tablespoon extra-virgin olive oil
Splash of chicken stock or bouillon
150ml half-fat crème fraîche
2 tablespoons chopped tarragon
½ tablespoon Dijon mustard
1 tablespoon lemon juice

1. Season the chicken breasts and heat the oil in a sauté pan. Sauté the chicken pieces over a medium heat until slightly browned and cooked through, about 5 to 7 minutes.
2. Turn the heat down to low and add the stock. When it starts to bubble, add the crème fraîche, tarragon, mustard and lemon juice and bring to a low simmer for about 5 minutes. Taste for seasoning.
3. I like to serve this with a portion of brown rice (about 40g) and a green salad.

Nutrition per portion: 330 kcal, protein 36g, carbohydrate 4g, fat 19g, saturated fat 8.3g, fibre 0g, sugar 2.7g, salt 1.25g

SUNDAY STEW

Dad made this very easy stew one weekend and it was delicious. As is so often the case, the quality of ingredients made a big difference. The stewing steak and the carrots weren't expensive, but came from a local farm shop, the steak was melt in the mouth and the carrots might have looked a bit knobbly, but were straight out of the ground and super sweet. Dad picked up the Parmesan trick from Nigel Slater and we definitely think it added something!

SERVES FOUR
2 onions, sliced
Olive oil
400g stewing steak (ideally from your local butcher)
1 teaspoon ground turmeric
1 teaspoon ground ginger
2 leeks, sliced
6 small carrots (Dad likes to slice small carrots lengthways)
400g tin of chopped tomatoes
1 litre vegetable stock (or enough to cover the meat)
End of Parmesan cheese (if to hand)

1. Preheat the oven to 150°C/300°F/gas 2.
2. Gently fry the onion in the olive oil in a casserole dish until translucent. Make room or remove the onion, add a little more oil and the stewing steak. Add the turmeric and ginger and slowly cook for 10 minutes. Lots of people like to sear the meat over a high heat so that it browns, but Dad takes it easy and the results are always melt-in-the-mouth.
3. Mix the meat with the onion, leek, carrots, tomatoes, vegetable stock and cheese, if using.

4. Cook for 3 hours, making sure there is enough liquid to cover the meat and veg. If at any time it looks dry, top it up with stock or a little water. You know it's done when the beef can literally be cut with a fork.
5. Check the seasoning and serve with your choice of green leafy vegetables. If you are no longer trying to lose weight, then add a couple of new potatoes each.

Nutrition per portion: 295 kcal, protein 26g, carbohydrate 18g, fat 14g, saturated fat 3.5g, fibre 5.3g, sugar 13g, salt 3.39g

SMOKED PAPRIKA AND SAUSAGE CASSEROLE

One of those dishes that tastes even better the second day! I know sausages don't sound very Flat Tummy, but I buy the little chipolatas and just have three per serving. I thought I'd include it as I devoured this meal even in the early days of losing weight.

SERVES TWO
1 tablespoon olive oil
6 chipolatas (herb ones are really nice)
1 onion, chopped
1 big or 2 small leeks, sliced
½ teaspoon smoked paprika
400g tin of tomatoes
Sea salt and freshly ground black pepper

1. Heat the olive oil in a wide-bottomed pan over a medium heat and fry the sausages for about 10 minutes until golden.
2. Add the onion and soften for 5 to 10 minutes.
3. Add the leek and soften, with the lid on the pan, for a few minutes.
4. Sprinkle over the paprika and then add the tin of tomatoes, with a splash of water (I like Nigella's little tip of using the empty can to swish a bit of water around and then add to the pot).
5. Season and leave the casserole to simmer very gently over a low heat for 20 to 30 minutes until the leeks are lovely and soft.
6. Serve with some green veg and your favourite healthy grain (bulgur wheat, quinoa, brown rice).

Nutrition per portion: 332 kcal, protein 16g, carbohydrate 18g, fat 22g, saturated fat 5.9g, fibre 4.8g, sugar 10.9g, salt 1.84g

✓ PORK MEDALLIONS WITH CELERIAC AND APPLE MASH

This is a comforting meal for when a salad just won't do, thank you. Pork fillet medallions are great because they come prepared as small portions and the celeriac mash is even more delicious than regular mash, or perhaps I am brainwashed.

SERVES TWO
¼ large celeriac, peeled and roughly chopped
½ large apple, peeled and roughly chopped
1 small onion, finely sliced
1 tablespoon olive oil
6 pork fillet medallions
A splash of white wine or vermouth
125ml vegetable stock
Tiny knob (10g) of butter (optional)

1. Put the celeriac and apple into a pan covered with water, bring to the boil and simmer for about 15 minutes, or until the celeriac is soft enough to mash.
2. Meanwhile, soften the onion in the olive oil in a heavy-based pan over a low heat for about 5 to 7 minutes. Transfer to a bowl.
3. Add the medallions to the same pan and cook over a low to medium heat for a few minutes so that the pork can brown a little before adding the onion back into the pan.
4. Add the wine and, after 30 seconds, add the stock. Cover the pan and cook over a low heat until the pork is tender – another few minutes. Make sure you have enough stock to reduce down to a nice gravy.

5. Drain the celeriac and apple, add a little butter, if using, and mash. Check the seasoning.

6. Serve up! I made the celeriac and apple mash as an experiment as I had leftover celeriac from making Hugo's Celeriac, Wild Mushroom and Rosemary Soup (see page 271). I thought it went pretty well with the pork and even had some leftover mash, which then turned into a bubble-and-squeak effort the next day.

Nutrition per portion: 332 kcal, protein 41g, carbohydrate 11g, fat 14g, saturated fat 3.1g, fibre 5.7g, sugar 9g, salt 1.72g

CUMIN AND CORIANDER MARINATED LAMB

Lamb isn't the leanest of meats, but at least that means you only need a little because it's full of flavour. This is another lovely weekend lunch idea from Caroline.

SERVES TWO
1 teaspoon coriander seeds
1 teaspoon cumin seeds
6 black peppercorns
3 cloves of garlic
3 tablespoons olive oil
1 lamb fillet

1. Grind the coriander, cumin and peppercorns with a pestle and mortar. Peel the garlic and mash it in with the spices and olive oil.
2. Rub the mixture all over the meat and set aside for at least an hour.
3. To cook the lamb you can either barbecue, griddle or grill it on a high heat for about 6 minutes each side if you like it pink, a little longer if you like it better done. Let it rest for a few minutes, then carve into thick slices.
4. Serve with Cumin Lentil Salad (see page 304).

Nutrition per portion: 365 kcal, protein 17g, carbohydrate 2g, fat 32g, saturated fat 9.9g, fibre 0.2g, sugar 0.1g, salt 0.14g

SWEET HONEY MUSTARD PORK CHOPS

Pork chops are not high on the Flat Tummy list, but when you can find little ones, they are such an easy supper. Serve with the Squashed Butternut Squash with Rosemary (see page 356), which is equally simple and always gives me a glow.

SERVES TWO
2 small pork chops
1 tablespoon honey or agave syrup
1 tablespoon grain mustard
A splash of stock
Freshly ground black pepper

1. Preheat the oven to 180°C/350°F/gas 4.
2. Place the chops in a baking dish. Mix together the honey or agave syrup and mustard and then smooth over the chops.
3. Add a splash of stock (I just use vegetable bouillon) and season with freshly ground black pepper.
4. Cover with foil and bake for 30 minutes, removing the foil for the last 10 minutes. Test the chops are cooked through by cutting into one with a sharp knife to check there is no pink and the juice runs clear.
5. I love this with steamed broccoli and mashed butternut squash with rosemary.

Nutrition per portion: 375 kcal, protein 24g, carbohydrate 6g, fat 28g, saturated fat 10.6g, fibre 0.4g, sugar 6g, salt 0.67g

VEGETARIAN CHILLI

This recipe is adapted from *Country Homes and Interiors*. I made this for a friend while staying with her and her two little ones. I was fearful of all the beans, but it was an absolute hit and so healthy. It takes a bit of time to pull it all together so make a huge batch and freeze some for when you don't fancy cooking, but do fancy a hearty meal.

SERVES FOUR

1 onion, chopped

1 fennel bulb, chopped

Olive oil

1½ teaspoons each of coriander seeds, fennel seeds and cumin seeds

2 cloves of garlic, crushed

2 pointed red peppers, deseeded and chopped

1 red chilli (or less if you don't want too much heat), deseeded and finely chopped

2 x 400g tins of plum tomatoes

½ tablespoon light muscovado sugar

2 tablespoons sun-dried tomato paste

400g tin of borlotti beans, drained

400g tin of flageolet beans, drained

2% Greek yoghurt, to serve

1. Soften the onion and fennel in olive oil in a large pan over a medium heat for about 10 minutes.
2. Crush the coriander, fennel and cumin seeds with a pestle and mortar and add to the pan with the garlic. Add the pepper and chilli and cook for a few minutes.
3. Add the tomatoes, sugar, tomato paste and beans. Give

everything a nice mix, bring to the boil and then reduce to a gentle simmer for about an hour.

4. Serve in bowls with a tablespoon of 2% Greek yoghurt or half-fat crème fraîche on top. It's perfect just like this for the full Flat Tummy effect, but you can always serve with rice or a jacket potato.

Nutrition per portion: 278 kcal, protein 13g, carbohydrate 36g, fat 10g, saturated fat 0.8g, fibre 9.2g, sugar 14.6g, salt 0.93g

VEGGIE CRUMBLE

With the abundance of vegetables around in the autumn, I adapted a Nigel Slater recipe for vegetable crumble. I remember when I was little we were often taken to a 'health food' café, the Harvest Restaurant (not to be confused with the modern-day Harvester). It was run by a hippy chef and I only realize now how lucky we were to have it in our little town in Dorset. This recipe transports me straight back to that café.

SERVES TWO

1 teaspoon dried porcini mushrooms (these are optional, but if you have them in your cupboard they add another layer of flavour)

Olive oil

1 onion, sliced

1 tablespoon rosemary or thyme leaves, finely chopped

1 carrot, roughly chopped

1 leek, roughly chopped

1 courgette, roughly chopped

100ml vegetable stock

Freshly ground black pepper

FOR THE TOPPING

40g breadcrumbs

50g walnuts, chopped

1 teaspoon pumpkin seeds (optional)

60g feta cheese, crumbled

1. Preheat the oven to 180°C/350°F/gas 4.
2. Soak the mushrooms in a little boiled water while you prepare the rest of the vegetables.
3. Heat the olive oil in a big saucepan and soften the onion

slowly for about 10 minutes. Add half the rosemary or thyme and continue to soften for a few more minutes before adding the carrot and leek and cooking for about 5 minutes.

4. Mix together the breadcrumbs, walnuts, the rest of the rosemary or thyme, the pumpkin seeds, if using, and half the cheese. Set this aside.

5. Add the courgette to the big saucepan. Drain the porcini mushrooms, keeping the liquid, and chop these before adding to the pan. Add the stock and the liquid from the mushrooms. Let it bubble up and cover for a couple of minutes.

6. Season the veg with black pepper and then transfer to a baking dish. Add enough of the stock from the pan to allow the vegetables to soak it up while baking.

7. Crumble the rest of the cheese over the vegetables and then add the topping evenly.

8. Bake for approximately 30 minutes until the topping is golden and crunchy.

Nutrition per portion: 462 kcal, protein 14g, carbohydrate 29g, fat 33g, saturated fat 6.9g, fibre 5.3g, sugar 11g, salt 1.74g

✓ SAM'S TURKISH MENEMEN

My sister used to make this when she first left home and it's another very easy one-pan supper that is bursting with flavours. Menemen is a Turkish fast food made of tomatoes, hot green peppers and eggs.

SERVES FOUR
1 onion, finely sliced
1 clove of garlic, finely sliced
2 tablespoons olive oil
1 or 2 green chillies, deseeded and thinly sliced
400g tin of tomatoes
Pinch of sugar
6 organic eggs
Freshly ground black pepper
A handful of any Mediterranean fresh herbs to hand
    (basil, oregano or thyme), chopped

1. Fry the onion and garlic in the olive oil for 5 to 10 minutes until very soft and starting to caramelize. Add the green chilli and continue to cook over a low heat for another couple of minutes.
2. Add the tomatoes and pinch of sugar and cook for about 5 minutes.
3. Whisk the eggs and season with lots of black pepper, then add to the onion and tomato and stir continuously with a fork over a low heat as you would with scrambled eggs.
4. Once everything is nice and fluffy, stir in the herbs and serve.

Nutrition per portion: 196 kcal, protein 11g, carbohydrate 7g, fat 14g, saturated fat 3.1g, fibre 1.2g, sugar 5.1g, salt 0.37g

✓ EASY VEG STIR-FRY

When I am in need of a vegetable boost, I throw this stir-fry together in a matter of minutes. I'll add some brown rice noodles or serve over bulgur wheat for a very quick supper.

SERVES ONE
1 tablespoon groundnut or vegetable oil
1 clove of garlic, crushed or finely chopped
½ teaspoon fresh ginger, finely chopped
½ orange or yellow pepper, deseeded and sliced
1 head of pak choy, rinsed and roughly chopped
A handful of button or shiitake mushrooms, sliced
A few splashes of wheat-free tamari sauce (a Japanese soy sauce)
A splash of mirin
Juice of ¼ lemon

1. Heat the oil in a wok and add the garlic, and then the ginger, cooking for a minute.
2. Throw in all your vegetables. The residual water on the rinsed pak choy will help to cook the vegetables nicely. Cook for a minute, then add the tamari and mirin and continue to stir-fry for a couple more minutes so that the vegetables are tender, but still crisp. Before serving, squeeze over the lemon juice.

Nutrition per portion: 155 kcal, protein 3g, carbohydrate 10g, fat 12g, saturated fat 2.1g, fibre 2.5g, sugar 6.1g, salt 1.06g

COCONUT AND SPLIT PEA DAHL

This recipe, adapted from one by Jane Sen in *Healing Foods Cookbook*, requires a bit of patience, like lots of Indian dishes, but is worth it and lasts for a few days in the fridge, so I usually make a big pot. Coconut is an interesting food from a nutrition point of view because officially it's a saturated fat, but many nutritionists argue that it doesn't act in the same way as other saturated fats. Personally, I subscribe to the 'everything in moderation' mantra and so while I love to cook with coconut on occasion, it's not something I eat every day.

SERVES FOUR

225g yellow split peas

600ml vegetable stock

2 tablespoons wheat-free tamari sauce (a Japanese soy sauce)

50g coconut cream

2 tablespoons olive oil

2 teaspoons mustard seeds

Bay leaf

1 onion, thinly sliced

1 teaspoon ground turmeric

1. Cook the split peas gently in a saucepan with the stock for about half an hour until soft.
2. Add the tamari and coconut cream to the split peas.
3. Heat the olive oil in a small pan. Add the mustard seeds and stir until they start popping (stand at arm's length).
4. Add the bay leaf and onion and soften for 10 minutes. Then stir in the turmeric and cook for a few more

minutes before adding to the split peas. Give everything one stir so the onions aren't too mixed in with the dahl.
5. Serve with basmati or brown rice (40g per person).

Nutrition per portion: 315 kcal, protein 14.3g, carbohydrate 38.9g, fat 12.4g, saturated fat 5g, fibre 4.1g, sugar 4.7g, salt 2.94g

CHANA MASALA (CHICKPEA CURRY)

This is a store cupboard fallback for me that takes zero effort and is perfect for a meatless Monday.

SERVES TWO

1 onion, chopped or sliced
1 tablespoon olive oil
½ teaspoon garam masala
½ teaspoon ground ginger
1 red or green chilli, deseeded and chopped (or ¼ teaspoon sweet chilli powder)
400g tin of tomatoes or carton of passata
400g tin of chickpeas, drained and rinsed
2 tablespoons of coconut cream

1. Gently soften the onion in the olive oil in a saucepan, adding the spices after about 5 minutes.
2. Add the chilli, tomatoes, chickpeas and coconut cream. Add a little water and simmer for as long as you can be bothered so that the flavours all mix and mingle, about 30 minutes.
3. Serve with a dollop of 2% Greek yoghurt either on its own or with a small portion of couscous, bulgur wheat or brown rice.

Nutrition per portion: 302 kcal, protein 12g, carbohydrate 32g, fat 15g, saturated fat 5.3g, fibre 7.2g, sugar 10.7g, salt 0.88g

RUPERT'S INDIAN STIR-FRY

I struggle to think of 'interesting ways with vegetables,' so thanks to Rupert for sending this recipe. Rupert says, if you don't like chopping onions because it makes you cry, drink some water, but do not swallow it down, let it lie in your mouth. It seems to work!

SERVES TWO
Olive oil
1 onion, finely sliced
3 cloves of garlic, peeled
Piece of fresh ginger the size of a small thumb, finely sliced
¼ teaspoon ground cumin
½ teaspoon coriander seeds
2 carrots, thinly sliced
½ head of cauliflower, broken into small florets
2 tomatoes, quartered
3 tablespoons natural yoghurt
About a tablespoon of chopped parsley

1. Gently heat the oil in a heavy frying pan. Put in the onion and let it gently cook for about 20 minutes. Take out the onion and set aside.
2. Heat up the pan a little hotter now and add the garlic, ginger, cumin and coriander seeds. Mix them around for a moment and then add the carrot and cauliflower. Now add the tomatoes and put the onion back in. Stir it all around so nothing burns.
3. After 10 minutes, turn off the heat, wait a couple of minutes and stir through the yoghurt and parsley, leaving a dollop of yoghurt to put on the top at the very end.

Nutrition per portion: 198 kcal, protein 9g, carbohydrate 22g, fat 9g, saturated fat 1.3g, fibre 6.8g, sugar 18.2g, salt 0.16g

On the Side

As a child I was extremely fussy when it came to vegetables. I remember my poor mum discovering them in my school uniform pockets because we weren't allowed to leave the table after lunch without eating up everything on our plates and I just couldn't do it. If there were peas on my plate, I thought the taste contaminated everything else that came into contact with them. But now I realize I was lucky in that my parents never forced the issue and gradually I would give new vegetables a go, so much so that now I ask for more cabbage and even carrots, which I firmly believed as a child I would never let pass my lips.

Now that I like, even love, vegetables, I am becoming more adventurous and finding new and interesting ways to cook with them. On many occasions I am perfectly happy with the simplest of side dishes – when the purple sprouting broccoli is at its best, all I need to do is steam it, add a tiny touch of butter and lots of freshly ground black pepper. For other times, it's nice to make a side dish something a bit special.

✓ HOME-MADE 'BAKED BEANS'

While tins of baked beans do contain some sugar, they are still a pretty good stand-by for a quick meal. These deluxe baked beans are worth the effort if you fancy something even tastier.

SERVES FOUR
1 onion, chopped
1 tablespoon olive oil
1 clove of garlic, crushed
1 tablespoon tomato purée
1 tablespoon tomato ketchup
1 teaspoon paprika
Sea salt and freshly ground black pepper
100ml half-fat crème fraîche
400g tin of cannellini beans

1. Sweat the onion in a little oil until soft, add the garlic and cook for a few minutes.
2. Add the tomato purée, ketchup and paprika, season and stir in the crème fraîche. Bring to the boil, then gently stir in the beans to heat through.
3. These are a meal in themselves with a small jacket potato or delicious with Cumin and Coriander Marinated Lamb (see page 336).

Nutrition per portion: 156 kcal, protein 6g, carbohydrate 17g, fat 7g, saturated fat 2.8g, fibre 3.9g, sugar 5.5g, salt 0.99g

BROAD BEANS

Broad beans are an excellent source of protein and a great reminder that we don't always need to include meat or fish in our meals. They also contain fibre, vitamins A and C, potassium and iron. Broad beans are a very typical Mediterranean vegetable – a Portuguese friend adds pesto to them to make a delicious side dish, which would also work as a main with couscous or quinoa. Another really simple idea is to serve broad beans with natural yoghurt, a drizzle of extra-virgin olive oil, lemon juice and ground black pepper. Health on a plate!

The top tip with broad beans is to boil them for a minute first in salted water, drain and pop into cool water. When they are cool enough to handle, remove the tough outer skin. They will then need another 2 to 5 minutes boiling or steaming to cook.

Cabbage two-ways from Goldhill Organic Farm, Dorset

I had to include a couple of recipes from my favourite farm shop in the world down in Dorset. Every time I go there, I can't help but exclaim at how firm the leeks are or how squeaky the beans and cabbages – the true test of freshness!

✓ CABBAGE AND MIXED PEPPER STIR-FRY

SERVES SIX TO EIGHT
2 tablespoons olive oil
1 large onion, sliced
6 sticks of celery, sliced diagonally (or finely sliced celeriac)
1 small cabbage, finely shredded
3 mixed peppers, deseeded and sliced
175g mushrooms, roughly chopped
Sea salt and freshly ground black pepper

1. Heat 1 tablespoon of the olive oil in a wok or a large frying pan, add the onion and fry over a high heat for a couple of minutes until beginning to brown.
2. Add the celery and stir-fry on the high heat for another minute, then lower the heat and continue to fry for another couple of minutes.
3. Add another tablespoon of olive oil to the wok, add the cabbage and fry for 2 minutes before adding the peppers and mushrooms. Cook for another 2 to 3 minutes until all the vegetables are tender, but still with a bite.
4. Season and serve.

Nutrition per portion: 96 kcal, protein 4g, carbohydrate 11g, fat 5g, saturated fat 0.6g, fibre 4.8g, sugar 9.5g, salt 0.59g

✓ CABBAGE DELIGHT

SERVES FOUR
15g butter
1 onion, sliced
1 small cabbage, shredded
½ thumb of fresh ginger, finely chopped
Pinch of sea salt and freshly ground black pepper

1. Heat the butter in a pan and soften the onion gently. Add the cabbage and ginger and let it cook gently until tender, but still with a bite. This will depend on how fresh the cabbage is and how finely you have shredded it, approximately 10 to 15 minutes. Shake the pan often to stop it sticking or browning.
2. Season and serve.

Nutrition per portion: 79 kcal, protein 3g, carbohydrate 9g, fat 4g, saturated fat 2g, fibre 4g, sugar 7.8g, salt 0.59g

RATATOUILLE

This is my even simpler version of ratatouille inspired by a recipe in *The Art of Simple Food* by Alice Waters, who runs the best restaurant I have ever been lucky enough to go to, Chez Panisse in Berkeley, California.

SERVES FOUR TO SIX
1 aubergine, chopped into 1cm cubes
Sea salt
Olive oil
2 onions, diced
4 cloves of garlic, chopped
A bunch of basil tied with kitchen twine
Pinch of chilli flakes
2 peppers, deseeded and diced (any colour you like)
3 tomatoes, diced or a 400g tin of tomatoes
Extra-virgin olive oil
Chopped basil

1. Toss the aubergine cubes with sea salt in a colander. Put a weight like a bowl on top and then leave the colander in the sink for about 20 minutes. Now, rinse well and pat dry (salting the aubergine means it will absorb less oil).
2. Heat about 2 tablespoons of olive oil in a saucepan and add the aubergine, cooking over a medium heat and stirring often. Once golden, remove from the pan and set aside.
3. Sauté the onion gently, adding just a little more olive oil to the pan if you need it, until lovely and soft, then add the garlic, basil bouquet and chilli.
4. After another couple of minutes, add the diced pepper and, after another few minutes. add the tomato.

5. Slowly cook the vegetables for about 10 minutes before adding the aubergine back to the pan and cooking for a final 15 minutes until everything is soft.
6. Before serving, remove the bunch of basil, stir in a little extra-virgin olive oil and plenty of chopped basil.

Nutrition per portion: 150 kcal, protein 3g, carbohydrate 14g, fat 10g, saturated fat 1.3g, fibre 4.5g, sugar 11g, salt 0.53g

✓ CHANTENAY CARROTS POACHED IN WINE AND THYME

Chantenay carrots are those dinky little fat carrots and are the perfect size for poaching whole. A friend tried these carrots at her friend's mum's house. She thought they were so delicious she immediately sent me the recipe. Thyme is thought to be particularly good if you have the start of a sore throat and the wine is clearly just for taste, rather than any medicinal purposes.

SERVES SIX
500g Chantenay carrots, rinsed and scrubbed
A glass of wine
About 10–12 sprigs of thyme

Bring a saucepan of water to the boil. Add the carrots, wine and thyme and simmer until the carrots are tender, but still with a bite, approximately 10 minutes.

Nutrition per portion: 30 kcal, protein 1g, carbohydrate 7g, fat 0g, saturated fat 0g, fibre 2.3g, sugar 6.2g, salt 0.05g

✓ SQUASHED BUTTERNUT SQUASH WITH ROSEMARY

This is a very comforting mash to replace creamy mashed potatoes on a cold day.

SERVES TWO

300g butternut squash, peeled, deseeded and chopped into rough 2-3cm cubes

1 tablespoon extra-virgin olive oil

1-2 teaspoons rosemary, finely chopped (according to taste)

Sea salt and freshly ground black pepper

1. Bring a pan of water to the boil and add the butternut squash, boiling until the squash is tender, about 7 to 10 minutes.
2. Drain the squash and return to the pan. Add the extra-virgin olive oil and rosemary, a pinch of sea salt and plenty of freshly ground black pepper. Mash to your desired consistency.

Nutrition per portion: 106 kcal, protein 2g, carbohydrate 13g, fat 6g, saturated fat 0.8g, fibre 2.4g, sugar 6.8g, salt 0.52g

BRAISED RED CABBAGE

As a cruciferous vegetable, all cabbages are high on the list of super veg. Red cabbage has an added intensity of phytonutrients, antioxidants that are good for general health and are specifically thought to be of help in the prevention of cancer. The apples add sweetness and cider vinegar is heralded by many nutritionists as helpful in the battle of the bulge.

SERVES FOUR

1 medium red cabbage, shredded
2 tablespoons olive oil
1 medium onion, chopped
2 cloves of garlic, chopped or crushed
1 large eating apple, peeled, cored and quartered
4 tablespoons cider vinegar
A pinch of sea salt and freshly ground black pepper

1. Rinse and drain the shredded cabbage.
2. In a large non-stick saucepan, heat the oil and cook the onion gently over a low-medium heat until soft, about 7 to 10 minutes. Add the garlic and cook for another minute before adding the cabbage and apple, giving everything a good stir.
3. Add the vinegar and seasoning. Put the lid on and simmer gently over a low heat for about 45 minutes or until the cabbage is very tender.

Nutrition per portion: 115 kcal, protein 3g, carbohydrate 13g, fat 6g, saturated fat 0.8g, fibre 5.4g, sugar 11.5g, salt 0.55g

GRIDDLED LEMON AND BASIL COURGETTES

Lemon, olive oil and basil, all Flat Tummy ingredients, combine in simple but delicious harmony to make the humble courgette a bit special on a summer's day.

SERVES TWO

2 medium courgettes, top and tailed and thinly sliced lengthways
Olive oil (for brushing)
1 tablespoon extra-virgin olive oil (for the marinade)
Zest and juice of ½ lemon
A pinch of sea salt and freshly ground black pepper
About 10 basil leaves, torn

1. Heat a griddle pan to a fairly high heat. Brush the courgette slices lightly with oil (or use an oil sprayer) and then griddle for 2 to 3 minutes on each side.
2. Mix the extra-virgin olive oil, lemon zest and juice and seasoning in a bowl and add the courgette slices, giving them a good mix.
3. Allow the courgettes to marinate for a few hours in the fridge before serving with the basil leaves torn over them.

Nutrition per portion: 127 kcal, protein 3g, carbohydrate 3g, fat 12g, saturated fat 1.7g, fibre 1.4g, sugar 2.7g, salt 0.5g

Bowl Food

Take your grain of choice, grill or steam a few vegetables, then layer on top of the grains and add a sauce on top. Or mix everything together, whatever you fancy. There is a restaurant in LA devoted to 'bowl food' and it's a great idea when you just want a simple, light supper.

Some of my favourite grains are bulgur wheat, couscous, quinoa and brown rice. For example, while it's asparagus season, a simple supper might be steamed or boiled asparagus, Spicy Tomato Sauce (see page 360) and bulgur wheat.

Bowl Food Sauces

SPICY TOMATO SAUCE

1 tablespoon light olive oil
½ onion, chopped
½ teaspoon mustard seeds
Pinch of chilli flakes
Sea salt and freshly ground black pepper
3 cloves of garlic, finely chopped
400g tin of chopped tomatoes
1 bay leaf

1. Heat the oil in a saucepan. Add the onion, mustard seeds, chilli flakes, a good pinch of salt and pepper and gently sauté for about 8 to 10 minutes until the onion is soft. Add the garlic and sauté for another couple of minutes.
2. Add the tomatoes and the bay leaf. Reduce the heat to low and cook for 30 minutes.

Nutrition per portion: 51 kcal, protein 2g, carbohydrate 4g, fat 3g, saturated fat 0.4g, fibre 1.3g, sugar 3g, salt 0.63g

ROASTED RED PEPPER SAUCE

This works well with grilled vegetables.

3 red peppers
Olive oil
Balsamic vinegar
Sea salt and freshly ground black pepper

1. Preheat the oven to 230°C/450°F/gas 8.
2. Line a baking tray with foil, slice each pepper in half lengthways and remove the stems, seeds and membranes. Put the peppers cut side down on the foil, brush with olive oil and roast for about 15 minutes until the skins darken and blister. Remove the peppers from the oven and keep covered while they cool. After about 10 minutes, remove the skins.
3. Put the peppers in a blender or food processor. Add a splash of balsamic vinegar, a couple of pinches of sea salt and a few pinches of ground black pepper. Blend until smooth and add more balsamic if needed to taste.

Nutrition per portion: 46 kcal, protein 1g, carbohydrate 7g, fat 2g, saturated fat 0.2g, fibre 1.7g, sugar 6.6g, salt 0.51g

✓ SALSA VERDE

100ml extra-virgin olive oil
1 spring onion, coarsely chopped
A generous handful of parsley
A generous handful of watercress
½ teaspoon sea salt
3 pinches of freshly ground black pepper
½ tablespoon freshly squeezed lemon juice
1 teaspoon white wine vinegar

Place the olive oil in a blender with all the other ingredients and blend until smooth.

Nutrition per portion: 211 kcal, protein 1g, carbohydrate 1g, fat 23g, saturated fat 3.2g, fibre 0.6g, sugar 0.3g, salt 0.64g

WHAT'S IN SEASON?

Spring has Sprung a Leek

With the spring comes a lighter touch in the food world. The asparagus are just around the corner and root vegetables give way to more greens and leafies grown above ground. It's a quiet time of year for fruit here in the UK as the last of the stored apples and pears are used up, but we can still rely on our southern European friends for lots of citrus fruit, mangoes and more.

Spring seasonal foods

Vegetables: broccoli, carrots, cauliflower, chicory, cucumber, Jersey Royal new potatoes, kale, leeks, onions, purple sprouting broccoli, radishes, rhubarb, rocket, salsify, spinach, spring onions, watercress, wild nettles
Fruit: lemons, oranges, passion fruit

Season of Plenty

During the summer we don't have to worry about food miles, there is an abundance of fruit, veg and fish on our doorsteps or just across the way in Europe. Here's a small selection of what you can find.

Summer seasonal foods

Vegetables: aubergine, beetroot, broad beans, carrots, chard, courgette, cucumber, fennel, leeks, lettuce, onions, peas, purple sprouting broccoli, runner beans, spring onions, tomatoes, watercress

Fruit: apricots, gooseberries, melon, peaches, raspberries, strawberries

Mists and Mellow Fruitfulness

Autumn is another bountiful season for foods that can be stored in cool dark corners throughout the winter months, from the apples and pears on the trees to the carrots, celeriac and swedes in the ground. Comfort comes with all the sweet vegetables like squash and pumpkin and make the most of the figs when they have their day.

Autumn seasonal foods

Vegetables: butternut squash, pumpkin, artichoke, carrots, courgette, kale, leeks, parsnips, spinach, swede, turnip, celeriac, beetroot, runner beans, sweetcorn

Fruit: apples, pears, blackberries, figs, damsons, plums

Winter Warmers

Root veggies and dark green leafies continue to be in season throughout the colder months, encouraging us to warm ourselves with hearty soups and stews. It's the time for nuts and spices and it's interesting that nature gives us the healthiest fats you can get (found in whole nuts) at this chilly time of year.

Winter seasonal foods

Vegetables: Brussels sprouts, beetroot, Jerusalem artichoke, spinach

Fruit: pomegranate, clementines, lemons, oranges, rhubarb, satsumas, tangerines

Other: sweet chestnuts, walnuts, mushrooms

Desserts

Puddings don't do a great deal for a Flat Tummy and so I haven't included a long list of them here. You can definitely have your cake and eat it, especially once you are back in balance, but the trend for pies and cupcakes is already rather well served in other books!

In many cultures, dessert is very simply fruit, the perfect amount of sweetness to round off a meal. I find it's really good to remind myself of that every so often; when you see a lovely ripe mango or melon, grab it and there's your pudding. I also like to have a couple of scoops of 2% Greek yoghurt with a little honey or, very simply, a strip of dark chocolate with a cup of herbal tea once I've done the washing up. On holiday, my friend made a fresh fruit salad with her treasure from the market: peaches, pears and melon. Simple and yet perfect at any time of the day.

✓ BAKED APPLES

A Flat Tummy Club member sent in this lovely message about apples in the autumn:

Before and during the war there was a huge push for people to plant fruit trees and orchards. So now we have a great heritage of fruit trees and you come across them every-where, not just in people's gardens, but along paths and on little patches of common. There is masses of fruit not being used, so get out and combine a bit of scrumping with a good walk for double the health benefits. When you've picked your apples, store them in a cool dark place and they will last for months (plus you can feed the birds in December and January and they will love you for it).

SERVES TWO
2 large apples
2 tablespoons raisins
2 teaspoons brown sugar
½ teaspoon ground cinnamon (optional)
10g butter

1. Preheat the oven to 180°C/350°F/gas 4.
2. Core the apples. Mix together the raisins, sugar and cinnamon and stuff into the holes, almost to the top. Dot the butter on the top of the holes and pop in the oven on a baking tray for about 20 to 25 minutes, or until the apples are just starting to fall apart and the tops look caramelized.

Nutrition per portion: 145 kcal, protein 1g, carbohydrate 27g, fat 4g, saturated fat 2.6g, fibre 2.5g, sugar 27.3g, salt 0.12g

ROASTED LATE SUMMER PEACHES AND FIGS WITH BAY

I remember popping to my local greengrocer to find some lunch one day and came back with a corn on the cob, a peach and a fig. 'What a lovely bit of lunch,' he said, and he was right. Roasting peaches and figs is the easiest way to turn an almost ripe piece of fruit into perfection.

SERVES TWO

1 peach, stone removed and halved
1 fig, halved
2 bay leaves
1 tablespoon runny honey
1 tablespoon natural yoghurt

1. Preheat the oven to 180°C/350°F/gas 4.
2. Arrange the fruit in a baking dish, tuck in the bay leaves and drizzle over the honey. Bake in the oven until the fruit is soft and gooey, about 30 to 35 minutes, depending on the fruit.
3. Serve with a dollop of natural yoghurt.

Nutrition per portion: 58 kcal, protein 1g, carbohydrate 13g, fat 0g, saturated fat 0.1g, fibre 1.2g, sugar 13.1g, salt 0.02g

✓ GRILLED PINEAPPLE WITH CHILLI AND LIME

It's difficult to tell living in the UK where they appear on our supermarket shelves all through the year, but pineapples are in peak season from March to July. A friend passed on this quick idea her whole family love on a warm evening after supper.

SERVES FOUR
8 rings of fresh pineapple, about 1cm thick
1 red chilli, deseeded and finely chopped
Juice of 2 or 3 limes

1. Preheat the grill or a griddle pan.
2. Scatter the chilli over the pineapple, along with plenty of lime juice, reserving some for serving.
3. Grill or griddle the pineapple for a few minutes on each side until starting to caramelize. Serve with a little more lime juice squeezed over at the last moment.

Nutrition per portion: 51 kcal, protein 1g, carbohydrate 12g, fat 0g, saturated fat 0g, fibre 1.5g, sugar 12.3g, salt 0.01g

DAWN'S BANANA LOAF

There isn't such a thing as a Flat Tummy cake, but when Dawn took up the challenge to create a healthier cake, her banana loaf won. I'm a terrible baker, but even I have had great success with this loaf, which is incredibly simple to make and is even wheat-free.

You can add sultanas to this loaf, which are very nice and make a good texture. The loaf is best served with a cup of tea or you can turn it into a pudding by adding a dollop of yoghurt and a splash of fruit purée. You can also cut and serve warm with vanilla custard, but we don't know of any slimming custards.

MAKES EIGHT TO TEN SLICES
200g wheat and gluten-free flour
2 teaspoons baking powder
½ teaspoon bicarbonate of soda
2 teaspoons ground cinnamon
75g butter
4 large bananas
75ml agave syrup or honey
2 eggs

1. Preheat the oven to 180°C/350°F/gas 4.
2. Sift the flour, baking powder, bicarb and cinnamon into a bowl. Add the butter in small blobs and rub in with your fingertips to make a kind of breadcrumbs.
3. Mash up the bananas and the syrup to make a purée. There can be some lumps as they add a nice texture to the cake.
4. Whisk the eggs, add to the bananas, and then add the mixture to the flour. Combine well and transfer to a greased loaf tin (21cm x 11cm is ideal).

5. Bake in the oven for 50 minutes, although do check often as baking times vary according to ovens. You'll know the loaf is done when a toothpick comes out clean.

Nutrition per portion: 209 kcal, protein 3g, carbohydrate 35g, fat 8g, saturated fat 4.3g, fibre 1.1g, sugar 15.8g, salt 0.55g

SOFT GINGERBREAD

Molasses is the by-product of sugar refining and so is far less sweet than sugar – the darker the molasses, the less sweet. The slightly bitter, treacly taste is perfect for gingerbread and means you can have some soft comfort without the usual refined sugar and butter that go into cakes. I also find ginger has a slightly sweet taste anyway. It's hard not to eat more than your fair share of this gingerbread within minutes of taking it out of the oven.

MAKES TEN TO TWELVE SLICES
250ml molasses
250ml buttermilk
1 heaped tablespoon ground ginger
Pinch of salt
250g spelt flour, sifted
1 large egg, beaten

1. Preheat the oven to 180°C/350°F/gas 4.
2. Mix the molasses and buttermilk together.
3. Mix the dry ingredients together, make a well and add the egg and the mixed molasses and buttermilk. Beat all the ingredients together lightly so that they are thoroughly mixed but still light and airy.
4. Pour into a lightly greased 23 x 33 inch pan and cook for about one hour, checking often as oven times do vary quite a bit with baking. The gingerbread is cooked when a toothpick comes out clean.

Nutrition per portion: 169 kcal, protein 5g, carbohydrate 36g, fat 1g, saturated fat 0.4g, fibre 1.1g, sugar 18.1g, salt 0.26g

DARK CHOCOLATE MOUSSE

This mousse packs a very intense chocolate hit so you really only need a small amount. If you're not keen on cinnamon, then add orange zest or try with a pinch of chilli. Dark chocolate is full of antioxidants and despite using milk instead of cream, this mousse has a creamy richness that tastes luxurious, but is only a tiny bit naughty.

SERVES THREE
85g dark chocolate
2 tablespoons green tea
½ teaspoon ground cinnamon
A grating of nutmeg
1 egg yolk
90ml boiling milk

1. Put the chocolate, green tea and spices in a food processor and blend to a breadcrumb-like texture.
2. Add the egg yolk and milk to the food processor bowl and blend.
3. Pour into three shot glasses or espresso cups and refrigerate for about an hour and a half for the mousse to set.

Nutrition per portion: 182 kcal, protein 3g, carbohydrate 20g, fat 10g, saturated fat 5.4g, fibre 0.7g, sugar 19.1g, salt 0.05g

PRUNE AND WALNUT COOKIES

This recipe is adapted from Jane Sen's *Healing Foods Cookbook*. Jane uses dates, but when I discovered they are high on the GI table, I tried using prunes instead. These are full of fibre, which we all need for a Flat Tummy.

MAKES ABOUT NINE TO TEN COOKIES
30g walnuts, finely chopped
30g prunes, finely chopped
1 banana, mashed
60g porridge oats
40ml olive or sunflower oil
1 tablespoon agave syrup or honey
1 tablespoon vanilla extract

1. Preheat the oven to 190°C/375°F/gas 5.
2. Mix all the ingredients together in a big bowl. Lightly oil a baking tray and spoon the mixture onto the tray (a tablespoon for each cookie). Flatten down the mixture a bit (the cookies will also flatten a touch while baking).
3. Bake for 15 to 20 minutes until golden.

Nutrition per portion: 108 kcal, protein 2g, carbohydrate 11g, fat 7g, saturated fat 0.9g, fibre 0.9g, sugar 5.9g, salt 0.01g

DARK CHOCOLATE BROWNIES

These aren't exactly going to help you lose weight, but as a treat they are at least half healthy with the dark chocolate, prunes and walnuts and they still had me oohing and aahing as I tried the first one warm from the oven. I have also swapped regular flour for stoneground spelt, which is thought to be easier to digest for many people.

MAKES ABOUT 10 BROWNIES
100g dark (70%) chocolate
50g butter
75g dark muscovado sugar
100g soft prunes
50g walnut pieces
2 eggs
1 teaspoon vanilla extract
70g stoneground spelt flour

1. Preheat the oven to 180°/350°F/gas 4.
2. Grease a baking tin (18cm square is ideal).
3. Break up the chocolate into pieces and add to a non-stick saucepan with the butter, broken up into cubes, and the sugar. Melt together over a low heat, stirring occasionally. Once melted, allow to cool for a little while.
4. Meanwhile, chop the prunes up finely. You may prefer to purée them, but I like the pieces of fruit in the brownie. Chop up the walnuts fairly roughly so that you have little pieces and slightly larger ones.
5. Beat the eggs with a hand whisk. Add to the melted chocolate mixture along with the vanilla extract and continue to beat until you have a lovely thick and shiny mixture.

6. Add the chocolate mixture, prunes and walnuts to the flour in a large bowl and fold in, mixing thoroughly.
7. Pour (or dollop) into the baking tin, smoothing the top with a spatula, and bake for about 35 minutes. All ovens vary so check every so often; once the top is firm, remove from the oven and allow to cool on a wire rack.

Nutrition per portion: 210 kcal, protein 4g, carbohydrate 21g, fat 13g, saturated fat 5.4g, fibre 1.9g, sugar 14.6g, salt 0.14g

7

Flat Tummy Workout

If, like me, you are not a regular visitor to the gym, but want to gently start toning your tummy, then try this very simple workout. At all times keep focused on your core and always use your tummy muscles for the exercises and not your back. You don't need any gym clothes for this workout; you can even do these toning exercises in your pyjamas! A yoga mat is helpful, especially if you have wooden floors. Remember that Flat Tummy Workout is just that; these exercises will tighten your tummy muscles but won't magic away any fat, that's where diet and calorie burning exercises like walking and running come in. Combine all three and you'll soon see and feel the difference.

Stretch

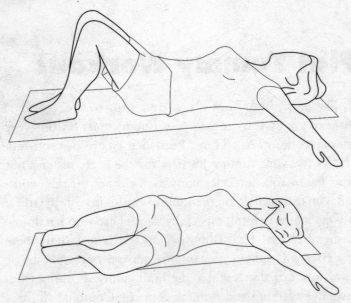

This is a very relaxing way to start and is a lovely stretch.

- Lie on your back with your knees bent, feet on the floor. The feet, knees and hips should be in line with each other and the head in the middle of the shoulders with your arms at a right angle to your body.
- As you inhale, gently roll your knees to your left towards the floor and, at the same time, slowly roll your head to the right, looking along and beyond your outstretched arm.
- As you exhale, bring your legs back up to the start using your tummy muscles. On the next inhale, roll your knees to the right and your head to the left.
- Repeat 4 times each side.

Crunch

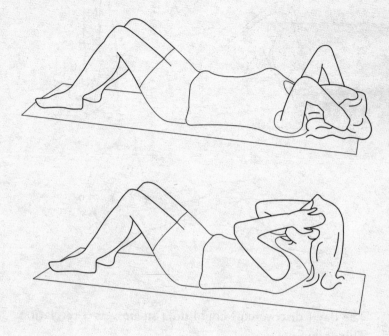

- Lie on your back with your knees bent, feet on the floor.
- Place your hands towards the back and sides of your head and keep your elbows pointing out to the side, rather than up to the ceiling, as you use your tummy muscles to 'crunch' and raise your shoulders up off the floor.
- Keeping your elbows pointing out makes your tummy work harder. Don't use your hands at all to move your head and don't strain your neck or your back – the key is to focus on your abdomen.
- Repeat for 3 sets of 8 crunches.

Sit ups

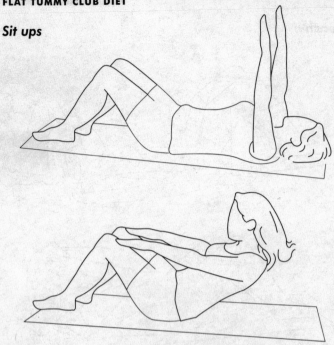

The day I discovered I could do a sit up was a revelation. This technique works!

- Lie on your back with your knees bent, feet on the floor and arms straight out on the floor behind you. Breathe in.
- As you exhale, use your tummy and bring your arms up and over at the same time to sit up. You have to believe it to do it, but once you have the hang of it, you'll know.
- Bring your arms back and lower yourself to the start position in a controlled manner, breathing in.
- Repeat for 2 sets of 8 to begin with, building up to 3 or 4.

Hundreds

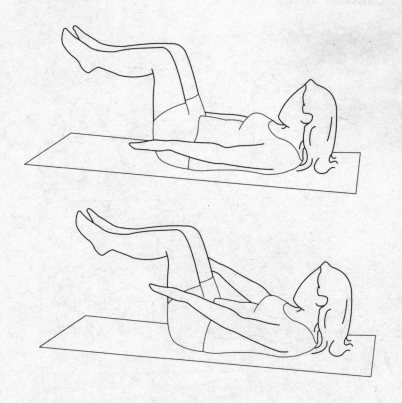

Lie on your back with arms at your side and your knees raised and bent at right angles so that your legs are 'floating' parallel with the floor.

Raise your shoulders up off the ground, engaging your tummy muscles as you would with a crunch, and then beat your arms gently up and down. The clue is in the name – the aim is to beat your arms 100 times, but start by just doing as many as you can and build up from there. As you get better you can lift your shoulders more which further engages your tummy muscles.

Crisscross crunch

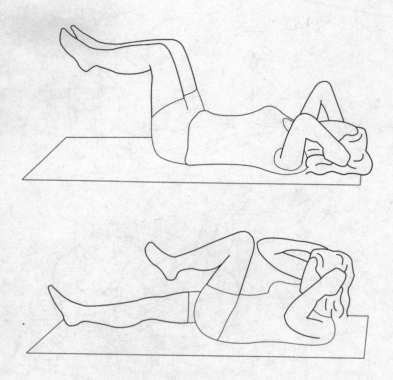

- Lie on your back with hands at the side of your head and your knees raised and bent at right angles so that your legs are 'floating' parallel with the floor.
- As you crunch, bring your right elbow to your left knee and at the same time straighten your right leg without letting it touch the ground.
- Now bring your right knee up to meet your left elbow and straighten your left leg. Keep up a continuous motion and go for 2 or 3 sets of 8.

Reverse crunch

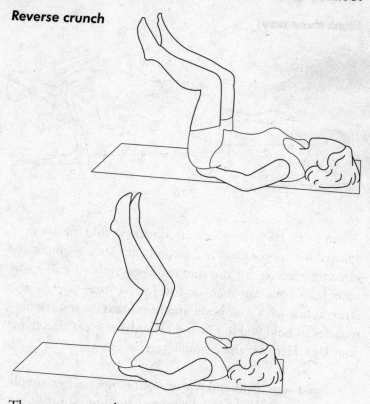

The reverse crunch targets the lower tummy muscles.

- Get in the starting position on your back with your knees pointing up to the ceiling and lower legs at about a 120 degree angle. You can put your hands under your hips to support them and help you to use your tummy, rather than your hips, for this crunch.
- Use your tummy muscles to pull your legs towards you and upwards. It's quite a subtle movement – you'll know it's working if you can feel your tummy tightening.
- Do 2 or 3 sets of 8, building up over time.

Plank three ways

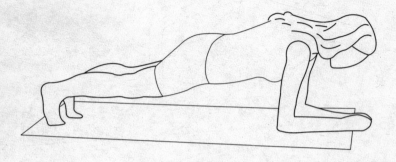

When I first tried the plank after a friend told me about it, I lasted for approximately 5 seconds! It's such a simple and effective exercise for the tummy. The key is to make sure your bum isn't too high or too low so that you form a straight line with your body, and then focus on your tummy muscles to hold you in position. It's also a great stretch for your legs. Here are three simple versions:

- Bend your arms and rest on your elbows. Then simply keep your body in alignment, holding yourself up with your tummy muscles for a count of 20.
- From the elbows bent position, bring yourself, one arm at a time, up to arms straight (the press up position), and then back down to arms bent. Repeat 10 times.
- This time turn on your side and again rest on your elbow, keeping the rest of your body straight for a count of 20. If you are anything like me and my friend Natalie, then you might shake a bit, but keep going!

Waist twist

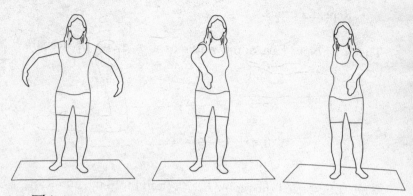

This is a nice exercise for your waist.

- Stand with your knees just slightly bent and hold your arms to your side, imagining you are holding a beach ball under each arm.
- Then gently swing your arms by twisting your waist, bringing your right arm to the front and left arm behind you. And then twist to bring your left arm to the front and right arm behind you.
- Do this slowly once, and then more quickly twice. Keep in mind all the time that you are holding the imaginary beach balls and try not to twist your hips, but keep them steady.
- Repeat 10 times.

Stomach vacuum

- In a standing position, exhale and then hold your breath as you suck in your stomach and expand your

ribcage. Hold for a count of 10 and then relax and
breathe in.
- Repeat 3 times.

That's it. Now have some water or a nice cup of herbal
tea . . .

RESOURCES

Exercise

Elanor Wallis-Scott is a personal Pilates trainer
www.zestforlifepilates.co.uk

Noel Smith is my Tae Bo Workout instructor
www.clubenergize.com

Darcey Bussell, *Pilates for Life*; Michael Joseph, 2005

Darcey Bussell, Pilates for Life DVD

British Wheel of Yoga www.bwy.org.uk

Nordic Walking www.nordicwalking.co.uk

City walking maps with 'calories burned' information
www.walkit.com

Stretch routines www.runnersworld.co.uk (search for 'guide
to stretching')

Fit Flops www.fitflop.com

Pedometers www.pedometershop.co.uk or
www.amazon.co.uk

Cycling equipment www.evanscycles.com

Look good exercising with gorgeous gym wear
www.sweatybetty.com

Food

Organic box home delivery **www.riverford.co.uk** and
  www.abelandcole.co.uk
Local food guide **www.freerangereview.com**
Brilliant seasonal food guide **www.eattheseasons.co.uk**
Grow your own mushrooms **www.suttons.co.uk/mushrooms**
Hugo's healthy catering **www.berwynevents.com**
Luzia Barclay's Herbs for Healing
  www.herbsforhealing.org.uk

Stress/Relaxation

Inner Space meditation courses and downloads
  www.innerspace.org.uk
Relaxation exercises
  www.patient.co.uk/health/Relaxation-Exercises.htm
Helpful NHS stress leaflet
  www.moodjuice.scot.nhs.uk/stress.asp

Cookbooks

Jo Pratt, *In the Mood for Food*; Penguin, 2008
Harry Eastwood, Gizzi Erskine, Sal Henley, Sophie Michell,
  Cook Yourself Thin; Michael Joseph, 2007
Cook Yourself Thin Quick and Easy; Michael Joseph,
  2009
Harry Eastwood, *Red Velvet and Chocolate Heartache*;
  Bantam Press, 2009
Anjum Anand, *Anjum's Eat Right for Your Body Type*;
  Quadrille Publishing, 2010
Susannah Blake, *500 Soups*; Apple Press, 2007
Jane Sen, *Healing Foods Cookbook*; Thorsons, 2000
Nigel Slater, *The Kitchen Diaries*; Fourth Estate, 2007
Nigel Slater, *The 30 Minute Cook*; Penguin, 2006

Alice Waters, *The Art of Simple Cooking*; Michael Joseph, 2008

The Greens Cookbook; Grub Press, 2010

Yotam Ottolenghi, *Plenty*; Ebury Press, 2010

Henry Dimbleby and John Vincent, *Leon: Naturally Fast Food*; Conran Octopus, 2010

Susan Tomnay, *Australian Women's Weekly 50 Fast Chicken Fillets*; ACP Publishing, 2004

Interesting Books

Michael Pollen, *In Defence of Food*; Penguin, 2008

Frances Moore Lappe, *Diet for a Small Plane*; Ballantine, 1991

David Servan-Schreiber, *Anticancer*; Michael Joseph, 2008

Muriel, Barbery, *The Elegance of the Hedgehog*; Gallic Books. 2008 (not really a food book but some wonderful references to green tea and the Japanese approach to food)

Gabrielle Hatfield, *Hatfield's Herbal*; Penguin, 2007

Elizabeth Gilbert, *Eat Pray Love*; Bloomsbury, 2007

Suzi Grant, *Alternative Ageing*; Michael Joseph, 2006

Brilliant Blogs and Websites

www.simplyrecipes.com

www.eatlikeagirl.com

www.skinnylattestrikesback.blogspot.com

www.jopratt.co.uk

www.well.blogs.nytimes.com

Apps

Epicurious (fantastic free recipes)

Whole Foods Recipes

Nike Training

Get Running by Benjohn Barnes
Men's Health Workouts
Canyon Ranch 360 Well-Being
NHS Drinks Tracker

Magazines
BBC Good Food (also **www.bbcgoodfood.com** and
   www.bbc.co.uk/food)
Delicious
Olive

ENDNOTE

I hope you have found this book helpful and it has given you some good ideas and the impetus to get started.

It's been a couple of years for me now and to be honest I feel like I eat loads and yet I'm staying at a weight and shape I'm really happy with. I think the difference is that I'm much more active and I make enough healthy choices to keep a balance. If I can choose a hearty soup for lunch rather than a toasted baguette filled with melted cheese and ham, then it's no hardship as I love soup and a baguette will send me into an afternoon slump, plus I'll balance it out with a treat I really enjoy at some point.

The earth shattering news is that, yes, the answer to long-lasting weight loss is to eat more healthily and exercise. But it's crucial that we find the means to fit these things into our lives in such a way that they are a benefit, rather than a boring pain in the oversized behind.

Here is my aide-mémoire that reminds me every now and then what Flat Tummy Club is all about:

Pre Flat Tummy Club

- Too much bread
- Too much booze
- Sugar
- Processed foods
- Cakes
- Pies and pasties
- Endless tea and coffee
- Mindless eating
- Overeating
- Sitting on the sofa
- Bad posture
- Feeling guilty
- Out of sorts
- Mood swings
- Can't be bothered

Post Flat Tummy Club

- Healthy breakfasts
- Soups
- Herbal teas
- Bags of seasonal fruit and veg
- Interesting grains
- *Real* food
- Lovely fresh fish
- Spices and herbs
- Delicious and adventurous cooking
- Mindful eating
- Eating just enough
- Walks in the park

- The endorphins from working up a sweat
- Savouring treats
- *Can* be bothered
- Feeling good
- Feeling in balance

So make a change and shout it loud or write it down. Get to know your own body and what works for you because we are all different. Focus on what you can add to your day, rather than obsessing about what you are giving up. Ultimately, I hope you will feel at ease with those foods you fear will send you into freefall and at ease with yourself. I'm not pretending it all happens in a day, but over time I've found the inner healthy me and as a result I seem to be a generally more relaxed and positive person. It took a big mental effort to get started, but I'm very glad I did.

I would love to hear your own Flat Tummy Club story.

Join in at **www.flattummyclub.co.uk**

Take care and good luck!

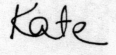

INDEX